The New DRCOG Examination

The New DRCOG Examination

Sample questions with explanatory answers

AALIA KHAN

BSc (Hons) MBBS (Dist) DRCOG DFSRH MRCGP (Dist)
General Practitioner, London

RAMSEY JABBOUR

BSc (Hons) MBBS DRCOG DFSRH DCH MRCGP (Dist)
General Practitioner, Gold Coast, Australia

AND

ALMAS REHMAN

MBBS DRCOG DFSRH DCH MRCGP (Dist)
General Practitioner, London

Radcliffe Publishing
Oxford • New York

Radcliffe Publishing Ltd
18 Marcham Road
Abingdon
Oxon OX14 1AA
United Kingdom

www.radcliffe-oxford.com
Electronic catalogue and worldwide online ordering facility.

British Library Cataloguing in Publication Data

A catalogue record for this book is available from the British Library.

ISBN-13: 978 1 84619 302 6

The paper used for the text pages of this book is FSC certified. FSC (The Forest Stewardship Council) is an international network to promote responsible management of the world's forests.

Mixed Sources
Product group from well-managed forests and other controlled sources
www.fsc.org Cert no. SGS-COC-2482
© 1996 Forest Stewardship Council

FSC

Typeset by Pindar NZ, Auckland, New Zealand
Printed and bound by TJI Digital, Padstow, Cornwall, UK

Contents

Preface

Following on from the success of our first book *nMRCGP Applied Knowledge Test Study Guide – Sample Questions and Explanatory Answers*, and as the format of the Diploma of the Royal College of Obstetricians and Gynaecologists (DRCOG) had changed, we felt that we were in a great position to produce another invaluable study guide.

We have found that holding the Diploma has enabled us to improve our clinical knowledge and made us more capable of providing a high standard of care in women's health.

In this book we have provided three full papers covering the entire DRCOG syllabus. They have been formatted as they would appear in the new exam to allow for practice under exam conditions. Furthermore, our popular subject index is provided to enable more focused revision of individual topics. Once again the explanatory answers have been fully referenced for your convenience.

Even though Ramsey ran off to the other side of the world, we had a great time writing this book across continents and hope you will benefit tremendously from it. Best wishes for the exam!

Aalia Khan
Ramsey Jabbour
Almas Rehman
April 2009

About the authors

Aalia Khan qualified from University College London Medical School in 2000 with a Distinction in medicine. She trained in obstetrics and gynaecology for three years in London before completing her GP training at the London Deanery. She achieved merits for all four modules of the MRCGP in 2006, gaining a Distinction, and was nominated for the Fraser Rose Medal. She was awarded a gold medal by the Ahmadiyya Muslim Community in recognition of her outstanding achievement in 2006. Currently, she works as a salaried GP in South London and lives in Surrey.

Ramsey Jabbour is currently working as a GP on the Gold Coast in Australia. He gained both the Diplomas of Obstetrics and Gynaecology and Family Planning during his VTS years in Maidstone, Kent. He achieved merits for all four modules of the MRCGP in 2006, gaining a Distinction, and was nominated for the Fraser Rose Medal. He is currently enjoying the comparisons and differences between different healthcare systems across the continents as well as gaining further experience in skin cancer medicine.

Almas Rehman graduated from the Royal Free Medical School in 2002. She wished to be a GP from that time and after house jobs gained a place on the Croydon VTS. She achieved a Distinction in the MRCGP in 2006. Currently, she is a GP in a busy South London practice and enjoys an interest in women's health and holds a letter of competency for intrauterine devices and subdermal implants. Furthermore, she takes an active part in teaching medical students, foundation year 2 doctors and registrars. In the future, she hopes to become a GP trainer.

Acknowledgements

Aalia: First of all, Alhamdulillah. Thank you to my husband Mashood for his support. And all my love to my baby Safa Maryam who taught me that it IS possible to be a mum, a working GP and an author, although it is not necessarily easy at the best of times! Thank you to my parents and mother in law and Muneeb and Shazia; without your prayers I could not succeed. I also want to thank Rezan Kadir at the Royal Free for always encouraging me to achieve my potential; she is a real inspiration. Ramsey if you want me to write another book with you, I won't do it unless you move back to England! Almas, what can I say, you are just as your name means – a diamond. I hope our friendship continues to flourish Insha'allah.

Ramsey: I dedicate this book to my Uncle Alan, who was such a strong and loving person in life and recently passed away. To his children, Ben and Lucy, our thoughts and best wishes are with you (I wish I was there). I would also like to give a warm hug, and a big thank you to my partner Ritu as well as my mum, dad and brother (Joan, Joe and Richard). Finally I would like to thank Aalia and Almas for all the hard work they have put in to completing the final touches of this book.

Almas: Alhamdulillah. Once again, Jazakallah to my parents for being so patient with me. Saba, now we can plan that trip Down Under – though maybe I should be in charge of the calculator! Sorry Zakir, I know you have set your sights higher, but house keys will definitely need to be put on hold for a while. Much love and salaams to Shakir, Hina, Ayesha, Sufyaan and any potential babies in the future, Insha'allah! G, hope you achieve all you wish for in life. Aalia thanks for putting up with my endless muttering/rambling and Ramsey, come back, it's not the same without you.

Subject index

(continued)

The DRCOG examination

The Diploma of Royal College of Obstetricians and Gynaecologists (DRCOG) is an examination that recognises a doctor's interest in women's health, rather than being a specialist qualification. To ensure that it is more relevant to primary care doctors, the format and content have recently changed.

Since February 2006, the candidate requires no specific training in obstetrics and gynaecology prior to attempting the examination. However, at the time of application, the applicant must hold provisional, limited or full registration with the General Medical Council or the Medical Council of Ireland. DO NOT be fooled into thinking this means the exam is any easier. The DRCOG examination is underestimated by many candidates and there is a significant failure rate.

It is important to understand that the examination tests both the knowledge of community *and* hospital-based medicine. It is naïve to expect that if you have done an obstetrics and gynaecology hospital post you will be able to sail through. Furthermore, do not assume that as a GP you will have enough experience to pass the exam without further study. However, it is straightforward and can be comfortably passed with the correct preparation.

EXAMINATION APPLICATION

The DRCOG is held twice a year in April and October. It is important to apply by the deadlines specified on the RCOG web site as late applications will not be accepted. Please read the web site carefully (www. rcog.org.uk). The candidate can indicate preferences for examination location, but the final decision of venue is at the college's discretion. The examination can be attempted five times.

The examination fee and registration details will need to be sent to the RCOG at the time of application and photographic identification will need to be provided on the day of the exam.

EXAMINATION FORMAT

The DRCOG used to comprise two parts: a multiple choice question (MCQ) paper and an objective structured clinical examination (OSCE). However, this has recently changed to ensure a fairer, more extensive coverage of the syllabus.

The examination now consists of 2 written papers:

Paper 1: 1.5 hours

Format	Number of questions	Marks for correct questions	Total marks	Recommended time (mins)	Percentage of examination
EMQ	30	3.5	105	60	30.0%
SBA	18 (1 from 5 answers)	2.5	45	30	12.9%

Break – 15 minutes

Paper 2: 1.5 hours

Format	Number of questions	Marks for correct questions	Total marks	Recommended time (mins)	Percentage of examination
MCQ	200 (40 five-part questions)	1	200	90	57.1%

EMQ – extended matching questions
These consist of a list of possible options for a variety of clinical scenarios. For each scenario one answer needs to be chosen. However, each option may be used once, more than once or not at all.

SBA – single best answers
These require one answer to be chosen from a list of five possible options.

MCQ – multiple-choice questions
These are traditional true/false questions with five-part answers.

SYLLABUS

The RCOG web site provides an extensive syllabus and curriculum for the exam. The following are the broad subject areas covered.

- Module 1 – basic clinical skills
- Module 2 – basic surgical skills
- Module 3 – ante-natal care
- Module 4 – management of labour and delivery
- Module 5 – postpartum problems (the puerperium) including neonatal problems
- Module 6 – gynaecological problems
- Module 7 – fertility control (contraception and termination of pregnancy)

You can access further information at www.rcog.org.uk

Useful resources

BOOKS

Baker P, Monga A. *Obstetrics by Ten Teachers*. 18th ed. London: Hodder Arnold; 2006.

Collier JAB, Longmore JM. *Oxford Handbook of Clinical Specialities*. 6th ed. Oxford: Oxford University Press; 2003.

Khan KS, Gupta JK, Mires G. *Core Clinical Cases in Obstetrics and Gynaecology: a problem-solving approach*. 2nd ed. London: Hodder Arnold; 2005.

Latthe M, Bath S, Latthe P. *Obstetrics and Gynaecology in Primary Care*. London: Royal College of General Practitioners; 2003.

McCarthy A, Hunter B. *Obstetrics and Gynaecology: a core text with self assessment. Churchill's Mastery of Medicine Series*. 2nd ed. Oxford: Churchill Livingstone; 2003.

Monga A, Baker P. *Gynaecology by Ten Teachers*. 18th ed. London: Hodder Arnold; 2006.

Nelson-Piercy C. *Handbook of Obstetric Medicine*. 3rd ed. London: Informa Healthcare; 2006.

Simon C, Everitt H, Kendrick T. *Oxford Handbook of General Practice*. 2nd ed. Oxford: Oxford University Press; 2005.

Toy EC, Baker B, Ross PJ, *et al. Case Files Obstetrics and Gynecology*. 2nd ed. New York (NY): McGraw Hill; 2003.

PUBLICATIONS

BMJ Clinical Evidence
British Journal of General Practitioners (BJGP)
British Journal of Obstetrics and Gynaecology (BJOG)
British Medical Journal (BMJ)

British National Formulary (BNF)
Drugs and Therapeutics Bulletin
Lancet

GUIDELINES AND WEBSITES
www.bashh.org
www.bpas.org
www.cancerreasearchuk.org
www.cemach.org.uk
www.cochrane.co.uk
www.ffprhc.org.uk
www.gpnotebook.co.uk
www.hmrc.gov.uk
www.nhlbi.nih.gov/whi
www.nice.org.uk
www.patient.co.uk
www.ranzcog.ed.au
www.rcog.org.uk
www.rsm.ac.uk
www.roysocmed.ac.uk
www.sign.ac.uk
www.statistics.gov.uk

Examination A
PAPER 1

EXTENDED MATCHING QUESTIONS

a Combined oral contraceptive pill (COCP)
b Progesterone-only pill (POP)
c Condoms
d Natural family planning
e Copper intrauterine device (IUD)
f Mirena® intrauterine system (IUS)
g Depo-provera® injection
h Implanon® progesterone-only subdermal contraceptive
i Sterilisation

For each of the following choose the most appropriate method of contraception. Each option may be used once, more than once or not at all.

1 A 17-year-old nulliparous woman who has irregular periods wishes to have a method of contraception that will also help her menstrual cycle.

2 A 47-year-old married woman who is having trouble with menorrhagia.

3 A 35-year-old woman who has a body mass index (BMI) of 38. She has mild learning difficulties and is having trouble taking her oral contraceptive.

4 A 38-year-old woman who is currently taking St John's Wort for mild depression and who smokes >15 cigarettes a day. Her mother had a hip fracture at the age of 50.

a Refer for ultrasound examination

b Offer ante-natal appointment at 42 weeks

c Refer for amniocentesis

d Refer for minimum twice weekly cardiotocography (CTG) monitoring and ultrasound estimation of maximum amniotic pool depth

e Refer for induction of labour

f Offer membrane sweep and refer for induction of labour

g Refer for once weekly CTG monitoring

h Refer for Doppler ultrasound examination

i Refer for assessment of risk of pre-eclampsia

j Expectant management for 24 hours

k Discuss options of managing an overdue pregnancy and offer ante-natal appointment at 41 weeks

l Refer for external cephalic version (ECV)

m Refer for Caesarean section

For each of the following clinical scenarios, choose one option for the management of common ante-natal problems. Each option may be used once, more than once or not at all.

5 A 28-year-old primiparous woman is seen in the ante-natal clinic at 40 weeks. She has had an uncomplicated pregnancy and is not in labour. Ante-natal examination is normal.

6 A 32-year-old primiparous woman is seen at 36 weeks. You hear the fetal heart above her umbilicus. Her blood pressure is 120/60 mmHg.

7 A 35-year-old multiparous woman with an uncomplicated obstetric history and normal current pregnancy declines the offer of induction of labour should she not deliver by term.

8 A 28-year-old primiparous woman is seen in the ante-natal clinic at 41 weeks. She has had an uncomplicated pregnancy and is not in labour. Ante-natal examination is normal.

a Reflexology

b Red clover

c Black cohosh

d Acupuncture

e Venlafaxine

f Combined cyclical hormone replacement therapy (HRT)

g Oestrogen only HRT

h Topical vaginal HRT

i Replens® topical treatment

j Clonidine

Choose the most appropriate treatment option for menopausal symptoms. Each option may be used once, more than once or not at all.

9 A 65-year-old woman has a new partner and complains of dyspareunia. She is hypertensive.

10 A 48-year-old lady has had to undergo a hysterectomy for fibroid induced menorrhagia. She is now suffering with significant hot flushes and mood swings. She has tried a few herbal medications and now asks you for a medication that is more likely to help her.

11 A 53-year-old woman, currently on fluoxetine for longstanding depression, complains of worsening mood and multiple hot flushes at night. She is keen for a medication to help her for this.

12 A 50-year-old woman is peri-menopausal and starting to have a few vasomotor symptoms. She is not sexually active. She is keen for advice on non-oral medication.

a Transcutaneous electrical nerve stimulation (TENS)

b Immersion in water during labour

c Entonox

d Intramuscular pethidine

e Epidural

Match the type of pain relief in pregnancy with the following statements. Each option may be used once, more than once, or not at all.

13 The most effective way of relieving pain in labour.

14 Shown not to reduce need for pain relief in labour.

15 Complications of use include delayed gastric emptying and neonatal respiratory depression.

a   Cefixime 400 mg oral stat dose

b   Topical imidazole

c   Metronidazole 400 mg bd for five days

d   Metronidazole 400 mg bd for five days, contact tracing/treat partner

e   Urgent gynaecology referral

f   Aciclovir 200 mg five times daily for five days, contact tracing/treat partner

g   Trimethoprim 200 mg bd for three days

h   Reassurance

i   Doxycycline 100 mg bd for seven days

j   Erythromycin 500 mg qds for seven days

k   Topical oestrogen

l   Oral antifungal treatment

For each of the following scenarios relating to vaginal discharge, choose the most appropriate treatment. Each option may be used once, more than once or not at all.

16   A 26-year-old woman complains of dysuria and an itchy, offensive vaginal discharge which is green/yellow in colour. She is sexually active. You notice strawberry spots on her cervix.

17   A 19-year-old woman's partner has just been treated for non specific urethritis (NSU). She complains of bleeding after sexual intercourse and a vaginal discharge. Her last period was two weeks ago.

18   A 30-year-old woman complains of an offensive vaginal discharge, which is not itchy. The pH of the discharge is >4.5.

19   A 22-year-old woman complains of non-offensive vaginal discharge that tends to change thickness every month. She recently stopped taking the oral contraceptive pill.

20   A 35-year-old pregnant woman complains of a thick, itchy vaginal discharge. You notice a curd-like discharge that adheres to the vaginal walls.

21   A 65-year-old woman complains of an offensive vaginal discharge and vulval soreness. There is no itching. You notice a bloodstained discharge from the cervix.

a Observe

b Serum beta-human chorionic gonadotrophin (ßhCG) level in 48 h

c Serum ßhCG level

d Transvaginal ultrasound

e Admit for intravenous antibiotics and intravenous fluid

f Immediate surgery

g Intramuscular methotrexate

h Repeat ultrasound in 48 h

i Serum progesterone levels

j Dilatation and curettage

k Take endocervical swabs and start empirical oral antibiotics

For each of the following clinical scenarios relating to acute abdominal pain, choose one management option from the above list. Each option may be used once, more than once or not at all.

22 A 20-year-old woman presents with lower abdominal pain and vaginal spotting; her abdominal and pelvic examination is normal. Her serum ßhCG level is 500 mIU/mL and a transvaginal ultrasound shows no gestational sac or adnexal mass.

23 A 30-year-old woman with a past history of pelvic inflammatory disease presents with a blood pressure of 60/40 mmHg, tachycardia, severe lower abdominal pain and guarding. A serum ßhCG level = 700 mIU/mL and the transvaginal ultrasound shows no intrauterine gestational sac.

24 A 24-year-old woman presents with a two-day history of nausea and vomiting, muscle aches and pain. Her temperature is 39.4°C and blood pressure is 70/50 mmHg. She appears confused and has a diffuse, sunburn-like rash. She has generalised abdominal pain, but her pelvic examination is normal. Her pregnancy test is negative.

25 A 25-year-old woman presents with crampy lower abdominal pain four days after being given intramuscular methotrexate for treatment of her ectopic pregnancy. Her vital signs are normal; she has no rebound or guarding on examination.

26 A 26-year-old woman complains of lower abdominal pain, recent painful intercourse and heavier periods. She denies any vaginal discharge and has no past history of sexually transmitted disease (STD). Her temperature is 38.6°C and on pelvic examination she has cervical excitation and tender adnexae. Her pregnancy test is negative.

a Rubella

b Varicella zoster

c HIV

d Hepatitis B

e Toxoplasmosis

f Cytomegalovirus

g Herpes zoster

h Syphilis

For each of the following clinical scenarios, choose one cause of infection from the list above. Each option may be used once, more than once or not at all.

27 A woman has just delivered a baby who shows hydrocephalus and diffuse calcification of the brain. She travelled to France just before she found out she was pregnant.

28 A woman went into pre-term labour and has given birth to a baby with thrombocytopenia and hepatosplenomegaly. On closer questioning she has suffered from a stillbirth in the past and remembers an ulcer on her vulva that resolved spontaneously.

29 A woman has just given birth to a neonate with non-immune hydrops and localised cerebral calcifications. She was not known to be unwell during the pregnancy.

30 A pregnant woman developed a widespread rash and fever at seven weeks gestation. Her baby is born with cataracts and microcephaly.

SINGLE BEST ANSWER: FOR EACH QUESTION CHOOSE ONE ANSWER ONLY

1 The Mat B1 form is documented evidence given to a woman who is in employment from a health professional showing the expected date of confinement. Evidence is acceptable if it is signed:

  a From the start of the 4th week before the expected week of childbirth (EWC)

  b From the start of the 11th week before the EWC

  c From the start of the 15th week before the EWC

  d From the start of the 20th week before the EWC

  e From the start of the 18th week before the EWC

2 Which ONE of the following statements is TRUE regarding vulval cancer?

  a It is a common cancer in women.

  b Women affected are usually under the age of 60 years.

  c Hypertrophic dystrophy does not pose an increased risk of developing vulval cancer.

  d 90% of all vulval cancers are squamous cell carcinomas.

  e Women with vulval cancer do not have an increased risk of cervical cancer.

3 With regards to complications of multiple pregnancies, which ONE is NOT TRUE?

  a Pre-eclampsia

  b Intrauterine growth retardation

  c Pre-term labour

  d Hyperemesis gravidarum

  e Pregnancy-induced diabetes

4 Which ONE of the following is TRUE concerning the treatment of menorrhagia?

    a Medical treatment must be carried out on all patients before surgery irrespective of uterine shape or fibroid size.

    b Medical treatment should be considered if uterine shape is normal or contains a small uterine fibroid less than 3 cm in diameter that is not distorting the uterus.

    c Dilatation and curettage may have similar results to endometrial ablation in the treatment of menorrhagia.

    d Tranexamic acid or non-steroidal anti-inflammatory drugs should be the first line of medical treatment used.

    e If a patient suffers from both menorrhagia and dysmenorrhoea, tranexamic acid is preferred over mefenamic acid as treatment.

5 What percentage of women suffers from diabetes in pregnancy in England and Wales?

    a 0.5%

    b 1%

    c 3%

    d 8%

    e 12%

6 According to the October 2006 National Institute for Health and Clinical Excellence (NICE) guidelines for urinary incontinence, for how long should a woman record a bladder diary?

    a One day

    b Three days

    c Five days

    d One week

    e Two weeks

7 Concerning the placenta and umbilical cord, which ONE of the following is TRUE?

    a A long cord >100 cm is associated with Down's syndrome.

    b The cord contains one uterine artery and two uterine veins.

    c A short cord <40 cm is associated with breech presentation.

    d At term the placenta weighs one-quarter of the normal neonatal weight.

    e A short cord impedes vaginal delivery.

8 Which ONE of the following statements is NOT true? The 1967 Abortion Act allows termination of pregnancy (TOP):

    a At any gestation if the fetus has serious abnormalities

    b At under 24 weeks' gestation if there is risk to a woman's life

    c At any gestation if there is grave risk to a woman's physical or mental health

    d At any gestation if there is risk to the physical or mental health of a woman's existing children

    e Over 24 weeks in an NHS hospital only

9 The risk of neonatal herpes infection from mothers who have herpes simplex virus (HSV) infection during labour is increased by all of the following, EXCEPT which ONE?

    a If it is the first episode of genital herpes

    b If delivery is by Caesarean section

    c If invasive monitoring is used

    d If maternal age is <21 years

    e If delivery is before 38 weeks gestation

10 Causes of recurrent miscarriage include all of the following except:

    a Controlled diabetes mellitus

    b Polycystic ovarian syndrome (PCOS)

    c Unicornuate uterus

    d Anti-phospholipid syndrome

    e Chromosomal abnormalities

11 What percentage of eclampsia occurs postpartum?

    a 5%

    b 10%

    c 30%

    d 40%

    e None

12 Which ONE of the following methods of contraception is NOT contra-indicated for patients with current or past history of breast carcinoma?

a COCP

b POP

c Depo-provera® injection

d Copper IUD

e Mirena® IUS

13 Which ONE of the following is NOT TRUE concerning risk factors for placenta praevia?

a Young age

b Smoking

c Cocaine use

d Prior history of placenta praevia

e Prior abortion

14 Which ONE of the following factors is NOT significantly associated with genital chlamydial infection?

a Age under 25 years

b In a relationship

c Using oral contraception

d Not using contraception

e Change of partner in the last three months

15 A 14-week pregnant woman presents with a history of being exposed to a child with slapped cheek syndrome. You request serology and the following result is obtained:

Parvovirus IgG-Negative

Parvovirus IgM-Negative

What should your advice be? Choose ONE option.

a Reassure – she is immune

b Give Anti-D

c Refer for intrauterine transfusion

d Retest in one month

e Refer for TOP

16 The most common indication for hysterectomy in the UK is:

a Fibroids

b Ovarian cancer

c Endometrial cancer

d Cervical cancer

e Postpartum haemorrhage

17 What is the most common direct cause of maternal death in the UK according to the most recent Confidential Enquiry into Maternal and Child Health?

a Ectopic pregnancy

b Sepsis

c Cerebral vein thrombosis

d Pulmonary embolism

e Eclampsia

18 A diagnosis of PCOS is supported by which ONE of the following?

a An FSH:LH ratio of 3:1

b A decrease in sex hormone binding globulin

c A testosterone level greater than 4.8 nmol/Litre

d A decrease in prolactin levels

e A combined total of 10 follicles in both ovaries

TVO7260

Examination A
PAPER 1 ANSWERS

EXTENDED MATCHING QUESTIONS

1 a

2 f

3 h

4 e

The COCP is taken in a cyclical pattern and therefore tends to cause a regular 'period'/withdrawal bleed every four weeks.

The January 2007 NICE guidelines for heavy menstrual bleeding state that first line pharmaceutical treatment of menorrhagia is a levonorgestrel-releasing intrauterine system (i.e. Mirena®). The added benefit for this patient is that if she is over 45 years of age and amenorrhoeic with the IUS she can keep it *in situ* until she is post-menopausal, which could be longer than the licensed five years.

In patients who have learning difficulties or who have a hectic lifestyle, long-acting reversible contraceptives (LARC) are a good choice. In view of this patient's high BMI the Depo-provera® injection is a poor choice as it can cause weight gain and the new guidance from the Faculty of Sexual and Reproductive Health on progesterone-only implants (April 2008) advises that there is no proven link with weight gain. The ease of use of the Implanon® is ideal for this patient.

The use of COCP, POP and Implanon® with liver inducing enzymes, such as rifampicin, carbamazepine and St John's Wort all have an UK Medical Eligibility Criteria category 3; that is, a condition where the theoretical or proven risks usually outweigh the advantages of using the method. The Depo-provera® is linked to possible osteoporosis so this should be avoided in a patient with a positive family history.

5 k

6 a

7 d

8 f

Women with uncomplicated pregnancies at term should be given advice on further management of a prolonged pregnancy: ante-natal appointment at 41 weeks for a vaginal sweep and a hospital induction appointment. If the woman declines, refer for increased ante-natal monitoring. This should consist of at least twice weekly CTG and ultrasound estimation of maximum amniotic pool depth. In practice, a GP would arrange this by referring on to the hospital consultant. Induction of labour is offered between 41+0 and 42+0 weeks' gestation. A malpresentation/breech/placenta praevia can all account for hearing the fetal heart above the umbilicus. Ultrasound confirmation is required.

National Institute for Health and Clinical Excellence. *Induction of Labour: NICE guideline 70*. London: NIHCE; 2008. www.nice.org.uk/guidance/CG070

9 i

10 g

11 e

12 d

This woman is suffering with probable vaginal atrophy. The most appropriate options would be a vaginal preparation in the absence of other symptoms. Furthermore, a non-hormonal preparation is always preferred, as there is a possibility of systemic effects with topical treatment. Replens® is a vaginal bioadhesive moisturiser.

This lady is looking for a more definitive treatment for her menopausal symptoms. Given her hysterectomy she is able to have unopposed oestrogens, which could control both her symptoms. Antidepressants would help with her mood, but may not have a significant effect on her hot flushes, and clonidine may be useful for her hot flushes but would do nothing for her mood swings. Some antidepressants such as the SNRIs (selective noradrenaline reuptake inhibitors) have been shown to help with some vasomotor symptoms.

Venlafaxine, a SNRI, is known to help with vasomotor symptoms and may be an alternative to fluoxetine. Twice-daily dosing is shown to be effective in short-term trials.

There are no studies showing a statistically significant effect of reflexology on peri-menopasual symptoms.

Royal College of Obstetricians and Gynaecologists. *Alternatives to HRT for the management of symptoms of the menopause. Scientific Advisory Committee Opinion Paper 6.* London: Royal College of Obstetricians and Gynaecologists; 2006.

13 e

14 a

15 d

Ninety-five per cent of cases have complete relief of pain. Complications include dizziness, hypotension, headaches, a longer second stage of labour and increased rate of operative delivery. It is not associated with an increase in perineal trauma, weakness of the pelvic floor muscles or long-term backache compared to other forms of pain relief in pregnancy.

NICE 2007 states TENS should not be offered to women in active labour due to research showing no conclusive evidence of its effectiveness. Bandolier shows evidence of the same conclusion.

Water births have been demonstrated to reduce the use of analgesia in the first stage of labour and support relaxation.

Pethidine is a CNS depressant with an onset of 15 minutes and duration of two to four hours. It is stated to have limited effect on pain relief in labour; however it does reduce anxiety. As it causes nausea and vomiting it should be given with an anti-emetic.

National Institute for Health and Clinical Excellence. *Intrapartum Care. Care of healthy women and their babies during childbirth: NICE guideline 55.* London: NIHCE; 2007.

www.medicine.ox.ac.uk/bandolier/booth/painpag/Acutrev/labour/AP001.html

16 d

17 i

18 c

19 h

20 b

21 e

Trichomonas vaginalis is an STD that causes an offensive green/yellow vaginal discharge and is treated with metronidazole. Don't forget contact tracing for all sexually transmitted infections. She should also be advised to have a sexual health screen. Strawberry spots on the cervix are rare.

NSU can be caused by *Chlamydia* and as she is not pregnant she can take doxycycline.

Bacterial vaginosis (BV) is a common infection usually by anaerobic organisms (e.g. *Gardnerella*), which causes an offensive discharge. The pH is altered in the vagina. Treatment is with metronidazole and to avoid irritants such as bubble bath. BV is not sexually transmitted.

Vaginal discharge does alter during the menstrual cycle and someone who has stopped taking the pill may notice a change and will require reassurance.

Candida infection is common during pregnancy (altered vaginal pH) and a topical antifungal agent is adequate. Don't forget to test for diabetes if it is persistent or recurrent.

You must refer for an urgent gynaecological opinion if a postmenopausal woman presents with discharge and bleeding. The cause may be atrophy requiring topical oestrogens, but the possibility of malignancy cannot be ignored.

www.bashh.org.uk

22 b

23 f

24 e

25 a

26 k

Serum ßhCG doubles every 48 h in normal pregnancy, A transvaginal ultrasound will not detect a pregnancy unless the serum ßhCG is above 1500 mIU/mL.

Most likely the patient has a ruptured ectopic pregnancy.

The patient has toxic shock syndrome, caused by an exotoxin of *S. aureus*, hence blood cultures may be normal. Risk factors include barrier contraception and tampon use. Skin changes develop from an erythematous sunburn-like rash to a maculopapular rash, then a few days later desquamation of the palms and soles. There is also conjunctival redness.

It is common for women to experience mild abdominal pain post methotrexate treatment; observation is suitable in the absence of signs of hypovolaemic shock or tubal rupture.

The patient has acute salpingitis, presentation may also be with right upper quadrant pain due to peri-hepatic adhesions (Fitz-Hugh Curtis syndrome). Blind oral treatment is with oral ofloxacin 400 mg twice a day plus oral metronidazole 400 mg twice a day for 14 days.

27 e

28 h

29 f

30 a

Toxoplasmosis is most dangerous to the fetus if contracted in the first trimester. However, transmission rates increase with increasing gestation. Hence, it may be more dangerous earlier on, but is harder to pass onto the fetus. It tends to cause mental retardation, chorioretinitis, calcification and hydrocephalus. Infection is usually spread via consumption of raw meats/pate and contact with cat litter. Remember to counsel pregnant women about the risk of listeriosis with unpasteurised cheese; the risk of vitamin A toxicity with liver and the risk of salmonella with uncooked eggs.

If maternal infection occurs before 8–10 weeks then congenital rubella syndrome is likely. This is characterised by heart defects, such as patent ductus arteriosus and mental retardation. Cataracts, glaucoma, retinopathy and microcephaly are also common.

Cytomegalovirus can occur in asymptomatic women. There is no effective vaccine and it is best to avoid contact with toddler's urine to help prevent infection transmission. Babies with cytomegalovirus (CMV) infection can have problems at birth such as hydrops, intra-uterine growth restriction (IUGR), chorioretinitis and microcephaly, or later manifestations, such as mental retardation, progressive hearing loss and visual impairment.

Syphilis can be transmitted via the placenta at any stage of the pregnancy and can cause miscarriage, stillbirth, polyhydramnios, hydrops, preterm labour and congenital syphilis. Affected women must be referred to the fetal medicine unit for regular monitoring of fetal well-being. After delivery, the baby should be tested for congenital syphilis, and treatment initiated if necessary. Other siblings in the family must also be assessed.

Features of congenital syphilis: Early (before age two years): widespread including gummata, condylomata lata, rash, haemorrhagic rhinitis, osteochondritis, hepatosplenomegaly, glomerulonephritis, haemolysis, thrombocytopenia. Late (presentation after two years): frontal bossing, teeth deformities, interstitial keratitis, Clutton's joints, saddlenose deformity, deafness and many more.

SINGLE BEST ANSWER

1 d
www.hmrc.gov.uk

2 d
Vulval cancer is rare: there are around 1000 new cases annually and it is the 20th most common cancer in women. Under the age of 50 it is rare. Ninety per cent of women will present with a visible lump/ulcer and 90% are squamous cell carcinomas. Women with vulval cancer have an increased risk of developing other genital cancers, particularly cervical cancer.
www.gpnotebook.co.uk

3 e
There is also an increased risk of antepartum haemorrhage due to abruption, placenta praevia, polyhydramnios, postpartum haemorrhage, malpresentation, cord prolapse or cord entanglement, twin-to-twin transfusion and malformations including conjoined twins.

4 b
NICE suggests the levonorgestrel-releasing intrauterine system should be considered as the first line treatment provided the patient is counselled as to the long-term benefits and advised to persist with treatment for at least six cycles. Other medical treatments include the COCP, norethisterone 15 mg daily from day 5 to 26 of the menstrual cycle and long-acting injected progestogens. Mefenamic acid should be used over tranexamic acid if both dysmenorrhoea and menorrhagia coexist. These treatments can be used long term or discontinued if not useful after three cycles.
www.nice.org.uk/Guidance/CG44

5 c

According to NICE guidelines for diabetes in pregnancy, 2–5% of pregnancies involve women with diabetes.

National Institute for Health and Clinical Excellence. *Diabetes in Pregnancy: NICE guideline 63*. London: NIHCE; 2008. www.nice.org.uk/guidance/CG063

6 b

Women should be encouraged to record for a minimum of three days their daily fluid intake and urinary symptoms. They should also try to cover a variation of days, which include both leisure and work days.

7 c

The cord contains two arteries and one vein. If there is only one artery there is an association with fetal anomalies, especially trisomies and cord compression. Normal placental weight is 400–600 g or approximately 15% of normal neonatal weight. A long cord is associated with an increased risk of fetal entanglement, knots and prolapse of the cord. A short cord is associated with a poorly active fetus, Down's syndrome, prolonged second stage, uterine inversion and abruption.

8 d

TOP is allowed under 24 weeks' gestation if there is risk to the physical or mental health of a woman's children. The other statements are all true. Termination can occur at any gestation if there is grave risk to a woman's life or her physical or mental health, or the abnormalities of the fetus are serious. Terminations after 24 weeks must take place in an NHS hospital.

9 b

Caesarean section does not increase the risk of neonatal herpes unlike the other four options.

British Association for Sexual Health and HIV (BASHH). *National Guideline for the Management of Genital Herpes*. London: British Association for Sexual Health and HIV; 2007.

10 a

One in 100 women has recurrent miscarriages defined as three or more loss of pregnancies at some point in the first 23 weeks. Diabetes and thyroid problems are factors in single miscarriages but when well controlled do not cause recurrent miscarriages. Uterine abnormalities (e.g. bicornuate uterus) are diagnosed with hysterosalpingogram and present with second trimester miscarriages.

11 d

According to the RCOG green-top guidelines, up to 44% of eclampsia occurs postpartum. Anti-hypertensive medications should be continued postpartum as even though blood pressure initially drops, it tends to rise again and cause significant morbidity. These medications may need to be continued up to three months post-delivery. If they are required longer than this, it may be due to underlying renal disease.

Royal College of Obstetricians and Gynaecologists. *Management of Severe Eclampsia/Pre-Eclampsia: RCOG guideline no. 10(A)*. London: Royal College of Obstetricians and Gynaecologists; 2006.

12 d

Current breast cancer has a UK Medical Eligibility Criteria (UKMEC) of four in all methods and past history within the last five years carries a classification of three. The copper IUD in view of it having no hormonal effects has a classification of one (i.e. condition where there is no restriction on usage).

13 a

Advancing maternal age, increased parity, previous Caesarean section, previous uterine infections or surgery are other risk factors. (Prophylactic use of antibiotics for Caesarean section, TOP and manual removal of placenta decreases incidence.)

14 b

Being single, not having children, leaving school early are other factors.

15 d

Current guidelines suggest retesting in one month because although the woman does not have a current infection, she is not immune either so may seroconvert. If the repeat sample is negative, you may reassure, but she is still susceptible. If IgG is positive and IgM is negative, she has been exposed in the past and is immune so you can reassure. If IgM is positive, retest the sample. If this is positive, refer for serial scans.

www.hpa.org.uk/cdph/issues/CDPHVol5/No1/rash_illness_guidelines

16 a

17 d

18 b

Blood tests should be carried out during the first week of the menstrual cycle and a diagnosis of PCOS is supported by:

- luteinising hormone (LH) to follicle stimulating hormone (FSH) ratio of 3:1 or more
- elevated free testosterone level
- low level of sex hormone binding globulin (can also be used as a marker for insulin resistance)
- 10 follicles or more per ovary
- raised prolactin level (40%)

A testosterone level of >4.8 nmol/L should prompt investigation for other causes of androgen hypersecretion, including Cushing's syndrome, and ovarian or adrenal gland tumours.

Examination A
PAPER 2

MULTIPLE CHOICE QUESTIONS

1 Causes of oligohydramnios include:
   a Bilateral renal agenesis
   b Posterior urethral valves
   c Post-term pregnancy
   d Prolonged rupture of membranes
   e Pre-eclampsia

2 Definitions.
   a Primary amenorrhoea is failure to start menstruation by 15 years of age.
   b Primary dysmenorrhoea is painful periods without identified organic pathology.
   c Menorrhagia is defined as blood loss of more than 80 mL in a normal menstrual cycle.
   d Secondary amenorrhoea is defined as absence of periods for more than three months other than when pregnant.
   e Precocious puberty is defined as puberty occurring in girls under eight years and boys under nine years.

3 Common causes of neonatal jaundice within 24 hours after birth:
   a Metabolic disease
   b 'Breast-milk' jaundice
   c Infection
   d ABO incompatibility
   e Glucose-6-phosphate dehydrogenase (G6PD) deficiency

4 Ovarian cancer.

  a This is the third commonest cause of death from cancer in women.

  b An elevated CA-125 has a specificity of around 80% for ovarian cancer.

  c The UK Collaborative Trial of Ovarian Cancer Screening (UKCTOCS) has found that screening with annual transvaginal ultrasound is just as effective as serial serum CA-125.

  d A risk of malignancy index (RMI) combines the CA-125 level, CT scan findings and menopausal status.

  e Ovarian cysts are more common in postmenopausal than premenopausal women.

5 Complications of ECV include:

  a Placental separation

  b Dehiscence of uterine scar

  c Precipitation of labour

  d Rupture of membranes

  e Cord entanglement

6 COCP.

  a The risks usually outweigh the benefit if a patient is over 35 years of age and smokes <15 cigarettes a day.

  b The risks usually outweigh the benefit if a patient is younger than 35 years of age and smokes >15 cigarettes a day.

  c Factor V Leiden is known to be an absolute contra-indication.

  d This may be used in patients with a family history of venous thromboembolism (VTE) aged <45 years.

  e This may be used in a patient with a personal past history of breast carcinoma.

7 Bishop's score includes the following measurements:

  a Station of presenting part relative to the iliac spines

  b Position of presenting part

  c Dilatation of cervix

  d Effacement/length of cervix

  e Consistency of amniotic fluid

8 Kleinfelter's syndrome is associated with the following:

a XXY

b Decreased libido

c Normal intelligence

d Tall stature

e Gynaecomastia

9 Epilepsy in pregnancy.

a Folic acid should be given at a dose of 5 mg/day.

b Stillbirths and fetal loss are twice as likely in epileptic women not taking anti-epileptic medications.

c Oral vitamin K for the mother may be required pre-delivery.

d Seizures are more common around delivery.

e Showers rather than baths should be taken.

10 *Neisseria gonorrhoea*:

a Is the third most common STD in the UK

b Is a Gram negative extracellular diplococcus

c Can affect the pharynx

d Is a cause of Reiter's syndrome

e Can be treated with intramuscular (IM) spectinomycin

11 Problems with breastfeeding.

a Mastitis can be caused by *Staphylococcus aureus* or epidermidis and occasionally streptococcus.

b In mastitis, breast feeding should be stopped on the affected side.

c Breast abscesses always need to be drained surgically.

d Sore, dry and cracked skin on the nipple area may be an indication of candida.

e Both mother and baby need to be treated for candida if either one develops symptoms.

12 Causes of menorrhagia are:

   a Hypothyroidism

   b Diabetes mellitus

   c Endometriosis

   d PCOS

   e Intrauterine contraceptive device (IUCD)

13 Concerning twin to twin transfusion.

   a This usually occurs in dizygous twin pregnancies.

   b This requires arterio-venous fistula between the twins.

   c In utero the donor twin becomes anaemic while the recipient twin is polycythaemic.

   d Post delivery, the donor twin usually requires the most attention.

   e Hydrops may occur in the recipient twin.

14 Prevention of UTI in women:

   a Increasing fluid intake

   b Complete bladder emptying

   c Passing urine less often (i.e. 'holding on')

   d Not to use lubricants during sexual intercourse

   e Washing the genital area 'back to front'

15 With regards to postpartum haemorrhage (PPH)

   a Retained placenta is the most common cause.

   b Oxytocin given with delivery of the anterior shoulder and controlled cord traction to deliver the placenta decreases the risk.

   c Asherman's syndrome is a rare complication.

   d Placental examination is important as a vessel in the membrane leading to nothing suggests a succinate lobe or retained placenta.

   e Putting the baby to breast stimulates oxytocin production.

16 Infertility may be caused by:

a Impotence

b Endometriosis

c Anovulation

d Retrograde ejaculation

e Tubal patency problems

17 Concerning placenta praevia.

a Patients with placenta praevia should not be given thromboprophylaxis, for deep vein thrombosis (DVT) prevention, as there is a risk of bleeding.

b Anti-D is not required for Rhesus negative women with Rhesus positive partners who have uterine bleeds.

c Corticosteroids should be used if pre-term labour or delivery.

d As per definition, pain is never associated with bleeding.

e Transverse lie of the fetus occurs in approximately 40% of patients.

18 Regarding TOP.

a Around 200 000 procedures are undertaken in the UK annually.

b Genital tract infection occurs in up to 5% of TOP cases.

c The risk of failure in first trimester surgical TOP is around 2 in 1000.

d At least one-third of British women will have a TOP by the age of 45 years.

e Women should be offered a follow-up appointment within a week after the TOP.

19 Components of the biophysical profile include:

a Amniotic fluid index

b Fetal breathing movements

c Gross body movements

d Fetal tone

e Reactive fetal heart rate

20 Bartholin's duct cyst:

    a Is treated by marsupialisation

    b May occur as a result of *N. gonorrhoea* infection

    c Is more common in postmenopausal women

    d May become a painful abscess

    e Appears as a swelling on the inner aspect of the anterior end of the labium majus

21 Causes of large-for-dates babies include:

    a Inaccurate dating of last menstrual period

    b Smoking

    c Post-mature fetus

    d Soto's syndrome

    e Familial

22 Effects of HRT:

    a High-density lipoprotein is increased

    b Low-density lipoprotein is increased

    c Triglycerides are decreased

    d Platelet count is increased

    e Creatinine level is decreased

23 Thyroid disease in pregnancy.

    a Women with pre-existing hypothyroidism will usually need to have their thyroxine dosage increased in pregnancy.

    b Maternal hyperthyroidism causes macrosomia.

    c 'Block and replace' regimes are a safe option in pregnancy.

    d Carbimazole does not cross the placenta.

    e Breast feeding is contraindicated in patients using propylthiouracil.

24 Fraser guidelines.

    a These apply to young adults under the age of 18.

    b The young adult must understand the medical advice being given.

c The doctor must ensure the patient understands the risks of not having any contraception.

d This applies if the health professional is not able to persuade the young adult to inform their parent(s).

e The young adult would come to no harm without the contraception.

25 Regarding maternal mortality in the UK, according to the most recent Confidential Enquiry into Maternal and Child Health:

a The maternal mortality rate is 10 per 100 000 live births

b >50% of the women who died were overweight or obese

c Epilepsy was the commonest cause of indirect deaths

d Most of the women who died after 24 weeks gestation delivered by Caesarean section

e Over 10% of the women who died from any cause declared that they were suffering from domestic violence

26 The normal menstrual cycle.

a Ovulation occurs at about day 18 of a 28-day cycle.

b Mittelschmertz is the term for mid-cycle pain caused by the rupturing follicle.

c The maturing follicle is termed a Graafian follicle.

d The corpus luteum starts degenerating four days prior to menses if pregnancy is not apparent.

e During the fifth month of intrauterine life the primordial follicles in the female fetus reach their maximum number.

27 Parvovirus:

a In pregnancy can cause fetal hydrops

b Is suspected if the cardiotocograph shows a sinusoidal baseline

c Is also known as erythema infanteolum

d Is infectious 14 days before the rash appears

e Affects around 1 in 200 pregnancies

28 Which THREE of the following are the UK centres for gestational trophoblastic disease?

a Southampton General Hospital

b Western Park Hospital, Sheffield

c Charing Cross Hospital, London

d St Georges Hospital, London

e Ninewells Hospital, Dundee

29 Induction of labour (IOL).

a This is usually less painful than spontaneous labour.

b This results in a higher incidence of assisted delivery.

c This results in a higher incidence of emergency Caesarean section.

d Around 1 in 10 deliveries in the UK are induced.

e Epidural analgesia is less likely to be employed.

30 Which of the following methods are used for home ovulation testing?

a Detecting the surge in LH

b Detecting the rise in progesterone on day 21 of 28 day cycle

c Body temperature on waking before activity

d Detection of 'fern-like' pattern in saliva by microscopy

e Rise in FSH levels in urine

31 Signs and symptoms associated with pre-eclampsia include:

a Severe headache

b Flaccid limbs

c Lower abdominal pain

d Visual disturbances

e Nausea and vomiting

32 Risk factors for ectopic pregnancy include:

a Depo-provera®

b Age

   c Caucasian race

   d Mini-pill

   e Pelvic inflammatory disease

33 Group-B streptococcus (GBS) carriage in pregnancy.

   a Routine screening for GBS is recommended.

   b Post-natal prophylactic antibiotics are not routinely recommended for low risk infants.

   c Early onset disease (EOGBSD) occurs within seven days and is less common than late onset.

   d EOGBSD tends to present as meningitis or a focal infection.

   e Intrapartum antibiotics should be used at the onset of labour and ideally within two to four hours of delivery.

34 Infection with BV:

   a Is the commonest cause of abnormal vaginal discharge in women of childbearing age

   b Is diagnosed using Amsel's criteria

   c In pregnancy is associated with late miscarriage

   d In pregnancy is associated with preterm rupture of membranes

   e In pregnancy is associated with preterm delivery

35 Human Papilloma Virus (HPV) immunisation in the UK.

   a This has been part of the national immunisation programme since 2006.

   b Girls aged 10 years are targeted.

   c Two doses over six months are required for immunisation.

   d Being immunised will not exempt women from cervical smears.

   e There is no national catch up programme.

36 NICE guidelines for diabetes in pregnancy, March 2008.

a Do not 'hand over' a baby born to a diabetic mother for community care for at least 48 hours post delivery.

b Admit to a neonatal unit a baby who is born before 34 weeks.

c It is recommended to feed the baby within one hour of delivery.

d Baby's blood glucose should be measured one hour post delivery.

e Metformin and glibenclamide can safely be used in breastfeeding mothers.

37 Turner's syndrome is associated with the following:

a XXY

b Tall stature

c Wide carrying-angles

d Webbed neck

e Right heart defects

38 Skin lesions in a newborn.

a Capillary haemangiomas are present usually after birth and grow larger before they disappear.

b Port-wine stains are dark and grow with the child.

c Cavernous haemangiomas are pale pink patches which fade with time.

d Sturge-Weber syndrome may be associated with port-wine stains in the facial nerve.

e Mongolian blue spots are blue patches on the buttocks.

39 Wilson and Jungner criteria for screening include the following:

a The condition sought should be an important health problem

b The method used to select those for screening should be reliable

c Facilities for diagnosis should be available

d There should be a suitable test or examination

e There should be an agreed policy on whom to treat as patients

40 Obstetric cholestasis.

    a Family history may imply a genetic connection with HLA-B8.

    b Itching, especially on the palms of the hands and soles of the feet, is a common sign.

    c Liver function tests are usually more than three times the normal value.

    d Ursodeoxycholic acid is licensed for use in pregnancy.

    e Women should not be allowed to use the Mirena® IUS post delivery.

Examination A
PAPER 2 ANSWERS

MULTIPLE CHOICE

1   T, T, T, T, T

Oligohydramnios is defined as a reduction of fluid surrounding the fetus, which is seen on ultrasound as a pool depth of amniotic fluid less than 2 cm. (Normal range 2–10 cm, fluid 400–1500 mL.) It is common in pregnancies that have progressed beyond term. Causes include failing placental function: placental abruption, twin to twin transfusion syndrome and systemic lupus erythematosus (SLE) causing immune mediated infarcts in the placenta. Maternal causes include: maternal dehydration, high blood pressure, diabetes, chronic hypoxia, drug induced (e.g. indomethacin and ACE inhibitors). Other fetal urinary tract malformations (e.g. cystic dysplasia and ureteral atresia) can also lead to oligohydramnios.

2   F, T, T, F, T

Primary amenorrhoea is failure to start menstruation by 16 years of age or 14 years of age if no breast development. Primary amenorrhoea can be caused by Turner's syndrome, cryptomenorrhoea, and Mullerian agenesis. Secondary amenorrhoea is defined as absence of periods for more than six months when not pregnant. NICE guidelines 2007 define menorrhagia as excessive menstrual loss interfering with either one of a female's physical, emotional, social or material quality of life (i.e. defined by the patient herself rather than quantitatively). Dysfunctional uterine bleeding is a diagnosis of exclusion and defined as heavy or irregular bleeding in the absence of recognizable pathology.

3   F, F, T, T, F

Metabolic disorders, red cell structure abnormalities and red cell enzyme deficiencies are all rare causes of jaundice within 24 hours.

More common causes include infections and haemolysis due to blood incompatibilities. Breast feeding is unlikely to cause jaundice immediately; it is more common for it to occur after two to three days when the natural body mechanisms cause a 'physiological' jaundice.

4   F, T, F, F, F
Ovarian cancer is the fourth commonest cause of death from cancer in women. CA-125 is the serum marker commonly used to investigate a pelvic mass; however, specificity is around 80% and sensitivity is 72%, therefore it is more useful when following up ovarian cancer for recurrence. The UKCTOCS (a large randomised controlled trial in postmenopausal women comparing TV ultrasound and CA-125 in screening for ovarian cancer) has not published any data yet; it has recently stopped recruiting. RMI combines the CA-125 level, ultrasound findings and menopausal status to give a more sensitive (92%) index of risk of malignancy. Cysts are much more common in premenopausal women as this group suffers from follicular or functional cysts most often. Ovarian cancer is more common in postmenopausal women.
www.patient.co.uk

5   T, T, T, T, T
Also if a woman is Rhesus negative, there is a chance that sensitisation may occur so all Rhesus negative women must be given Anti-D if undergoing ECV.

6   F, F, T, T, T
UK Medical Eligibility Criteria can be found on the Faculty of Sexual and Reproductive Health web site.
www.ffprhc.org.uk

This identifies the risks/benefits for each contraceptive method.
- UKMEC 1 – the method can be used without restriction
- UKMEC 2 – the method's advantages generally outweigh any risks
- UKMEC 3 – the method's risks usually outweigh the advantages
- UKMEC 4 – represents an unacceptable health risk
- UKMEC 3:
    —over 35 years old and smoke <15/day

—a first degree relative with a history of VTE at age <45, but UKMEC 2 if >45 years

—past history and over 5 years of no active breast cancer

- UKMEC 4:

—over 35 years old and smokes >15/day

—any known thrombogenic mutation

Remember that UKMEC 3 methods can be used if the other methods are unacceptable or unsuitable. The patient's risk of pregnancy and all of its consequences must be taken into consideration and discussed at length with the patient. It may be appropriate to refer to a specialist in these situations.

7 F, F, T, T, F

Bishop's score is used to assess favourability of the cervix and is reached by performing a vaginal examination and noting the following cervical features:

	Score			
Cervical feature	0	1	2	3
Dilatation (cm)	0	1–2	3–4	5–6
% effacement	0–30	40–60	60–70	80+
Station of presenting part relative to ischial spines (cm)	−3	−2	−1/0	+1/+2
Consistency	Firm	Medium	Soft	–
Position	Posterior	Mid-position	Anterior	–

Bishop EH. Pelvic scoring for elective induction. *Obstet Gynecol.* 1964; **24**(2): 266–8.

8 T, T, F, T, T

This is the commonest cause of male hypogonadism. It is associated with low IQ and either complete failure of sexual maturation or very little maturation. The arm span may exceed the length of the body.

9 T, T, T, T, T

Twelve weeks preconceptual 5 mg folic acid daily to reduce the risk of neural tube defects, which should be continued until at least the end of the first trimester; however, some doctors counsel taking it throughout pregnancy. Even if a woman is not taking medications the rate of stillbirths and fetal loss is high. Epileptic women taking hepatic enzyme-inducing drugs should take oral vitamin K in the last four weeks of pregnancy to reduce the risk of haemorrhagic disease of the newborn. Showering rather than taking baths is recommended as seizure frequency may increase. Serial drug levels are only necessary in those women whose epilepsy is uncontrolled or if dosages are being changed. A baseline drug level is prudent if serial doses are contemplated in future. Ante-natal care should take place in joint obstetric/ neurology or obstetric medicine clinic. Pre-conceptual discussion should take place with the GP well before pregnancy is contemplated and referral to an epilepsy pre-conceptual clinic is advised. Best chances of success with planned pregnancy to allow time for seizure control and drug regimen changes. Worst scenario is of woman who presents once pregnant and is on a drug that may cause defects; stops taking drugs and puts herself/fetus at risk of further morbidity/ mortality. Tuberous sclerosis, neurofibromatosis and other myoclonic conditions are associated with epilepsy.

Nelson-Piercy C. *Handbook of Obstetric Medicine*. 2nd ed. London: Martin Dunitz; 2002.

Epilepsy Guidelines Group. *Primary Care Guidelines for the Management of Females with Epilepsy*. London: The Royal Society of Medicine Press Ltd; 2004.

10 F, F, T, F, T

N. gonorrhoea, a Gram negative intracellular diplococcus, is the second most common STD in the UK. It frequently presents asymptomatically (50%), but other features include vaginal discharge (common), lower abdominal pain and, more rarely, intermenstrual bleeding. It can affect the mucous membranes of the pharynx, cervix, conjunctiva, anus and urethra. Complications include pelvic inflammatory disease. Reiter's syndrome is by definition a triad of non-gonococcal urethritis, arthritis and conjunctivitis. Treatment regimen according to the British Association of Sexual Health and HIV is a single dose of IM ceftriaxone, IM cefixime or IM spectinomycin. Oral alternative regimens are used where prevalence is low or antibiotic sensitivity has been confirmed. Patients with confirmed infection should see a health advisor in an STD clinic to ensure correct contact tracing. Test of cure is no longer recommended if asymptomatic and treatment regimen is completed.

www.bashh.org

11 T, F, F, T, T

Mastitis can be treated empirically with flucloxacillin as it has good coverage for staphylococcus. The mother should be encouraged to feed from the affected breast as this will encourage drainage of milk from the affected segment. However, if this is too painful the other breast may be offered to the baby and the affected side may need to be expressed. Candida is very difficult to diagnose, but the diagnosis can be pretty reliably made with a combination of skin soreness, burning pain, stabbing pain or skin changes, which include flaky or shiny skin (1). The mother should be treated with topical creams such as miconazole and the baby should also be treated, for example, with nystatin drops. If only one is treated both parties will continue to pass the infection between them. It is important to review a diagnosis if the symptoms are not settling; don't forget, breast cancer can present in pregnancy and in the postpartum period.

Francis-Morrill J, Heinig MJ, Pappagianis D, *et al*. Diagnostic value of signs and symptoms of mammary candidosis among lactating women. *J Hum Lact*. 2004; **20**(3): 288–95.

12 T, F, T, F, T

Other causes of menorrhagia include pelvic inflammatory disease (PID), endometrial hypoplasia, uterine fibroids, clotting disorders (e.g. von Willebrand's disease), psychosomatic disturbances, drugs (e.g. misoprostol) or anticoagulation therapy. PCOS causes oligomenorrhea and diabetes mellitus has no effect on menstruation.

13 F, T, T, F, T

Only occurs in monozygotic monochorionic pregnancies; however, they may be mono or diamniotic. The donor may also show growth retardation (with birth weight usually 20% less than the recipient), anaemia, hypobilirubinaemia. The recipient may have hypertension, hypoglycaemia, hypocalcaemia, hyperbilirubinaemia, macrosomia, cardiac failure, and if severe, hydrops. An extreme form is termed 'stuck on syndrome', where there is no fluid around the donor twin (anhydramnios) and polyhydramnios around the recipient. Post delivery, the recipient twin needs the most care and attention as it may be suffering from fluid overload, polycythemia and hyperviscosity syndrome.

14 T, T, F, F, F

It is important to drink a large amount of water, pass urine frequently and to ensure complete bladder emptying. These measures will prevent a significant number of UTIs. There is more chance of a UTI occurring on 'old', concentrated urine, which has sat in the bladder for some length of time. Washing before and after sexual intercourse prevents UTIs as does washing 'front to back' as there is less likelihood of bacteria passing forward from around the anal margins. Lubrication is important as it is less likely to cause trauma to the vaginal tracts.

15 F, T, F, T, T
The most common cause is uterine atony (90%); other causes include retained placenta, soft tissue laceration, uterine inversion and coagulation disorder (e.g. von Willebrand's disease). Sheehan's syndrome is pituitary infarction (usually anterior but rarely posterior as well) due to severe obstetric shock and PPH occurring in approximately 1 in 10 000 pregnancies.

16 T, T, T, T, T
Semen quality provides 40% of causes of infertility, ovulatory disorders 30% and tubal problems 30%. However, there are still a proportion of cases where no obvious cause can be found.

17 F, F, T, F, F
In 25% of cases spontaneous labour occurs in the next few days after a bleed. In 10% of cases there is some initial pain with placenta praevia. In 15% of cases the fetus presents as transverse or oblique. Thromboprophylaxis is indicated if increased risk of thromboembolism when the mother is managed in hospital and unfractionated heparin should be used over longer acting enoxaparin. Major placenta praevia covers the cervical os as compared to minor that does not. Transvaginal ultrasound is safe in placenta praevia and is more accurate than abdominal ultrasound for locating the placenta. Placental migration is less likely if the mother has had a previous Caesarean section or has a posterior lying placenta.

18 T, F, T, T, F
Genital tract infection occurs in up to 10% of cases, and is reduced by screening and antibiotic prophylaxis. Women should be offered a follow up appointment within two weeks, either at the place of procedure or with the referring clinician.

Royal College of Obstetricians and Gynaecologists. *The Care of Women Requesting Induced Abortion: green-top* 7. London: Royal College of Obstetricians and Gynaecologists; 2004.

www.rcog.org.uk/files/rcog-corp/uploaded-files/NEBInduced Abortionfull.pdf

19 T, T, T, T, T

It is a non invasive method requiring ultrasound to determine the fetal wellbeing. Each of the five components is given 2 points if normal or 0 if abnormal. Scores of greater than 8 are normal, 4–6 equivocal, and below 4 is abnormal, which may indicate the need for immediate delivery.

20 T, T, F, T, F

A Bartholin's cyst can occur if the duct gets blocked, causing a swelling on the inner aspect of the posterior end of the labium majus. Infection can cause a painful abscess. Treatment is by marsupialising the cyst: incising the cyst and suturing its lining epithelium to the skin to form a small sinus. However recurrence can occur and excision of the cyst may be necessary. *N. gonorrhoea* or *Chlamydia* may be the cause. Bartholin's cyst is more common in women aged 20–30 years.

21 T, F, F, T, T

Large-for-dates is a baby whose birth weight, when plotted against a growth chart of body weight and gestational age, is demonstrated to be over the 90th centile. Also, maternal diabetes, chromosomal defects, hydrops fetalis and Beckwith Wiedemann syndrome are possible causes. Post-mature fetuses are not usually large because placental insufficiency slows the rate of growth.

22 T, F, F, F, F

HRT has a tendency to increase high-density lipoprotein (HDL) and decrease low-density lipoprotein (LDL) levels. Triglycerides are increased. There is no known effect on platelets even though there is an overall increased risk of venous thromboembolic events with HRT. This increased risk of VTE is especially apparent within the first two years of starting HRT. There is no effect on renal function.

www.nhlbi.nih.gov/whi/

23 T, F, F, F, F

Both hypothyroidism and hyperthyroidism can be difficult to detect in pregnancy and both require close monitoring of thyroid function test throughout the pregnancy. Women who have hypothyroidism prior to the pregnancy will usually require an increased dosage. Maternal hyperthyroidism is usually caused by Grave's disease and can cause low birth weight, preterm labour and increased perinatal mortality. Both carbimazole and propylthiouracil cross the placenta and can cause transient hypothyroidism in the neonate. Breast feeding is allowed with both of these medications. 'Block and replace' regimes, such as those using radioactive iodine, are contra-indicated as they will irreversibly damage the fetal thyroid tissue also.

24 F, T, T, T, F

The Fraser guidelines were laid out after the case of Gillick v West Norfolk and Wisbech AHA and DHSS in 1985. Lord Fraser deemed the guidelines necessary to aid health professionals in this very difficult subject of contraception for those aged younger than 16 years. If it is felt that the young adult would have sexual relations without contraception and thus come to potential harm rather than discuss it with their parents, then it is in their best interests to treat them, to keep them safe from unwanted pregnancies.

25 F, T, F, T, T

The UK maternal mortality rate is 13.95 per 100 000 maternities. Maternities are defined as the number of pregnancies resulting in a registered live birth at any gestation or registered stillbirth. The effect of obesity cannot be ignored. Cardiac disease was the commonest cause of indirect deaths and the commonest cause of overall deaths. Domestic violence is common and increases the risk of maternal mortality. Women should always be screened at booking for risk of domestic violence.

Lewis G (editor). *Saving mothers' lives: reviewing maternal deaths to make motherhood safer: 2003–2005. The Seventh Report on Confidential Enquiries into Maternal Deaths in the United Kingdom.* London: The Confidential Enquiry into Maternal and Child Health (CEMACH); 2007.

26 F, T, T, T, T

Uterine cycle is split into three phases:

- Proliferative – increasing thickness of endometrial lining from 0.5 mm to between 3.5 and 5 mm.
- Secretory – endometrium becoming more vascular and glandular, stimulated by oestrogen and progesterone from the corpus luteum.
- Menstrual phase – regression of the corpus luteum and subsequent decrease in hormones lends to necrosis of the endometrium with subsequent bleeding.

The menstrual cycle starts with several primordial follicles enlarging, stimulated by FSH. Normally one follicle becomes dominant producing inhibin, leading to atresia of the other follicles. Cells within this dominant structure also produce a marked increase in oestrogen, which leads to a surge in LH. This mid-cycle surge in LH leads to ovulation. After rupturing, the corpus luteum secretes both progesterone and oestrogen. The production of progesterone distinguishes the luteal from the follicular phase. Progesterone prepares the endometrium for implantation and suppression in growth of other new follicles.

27 T, T, F, F, F
Parvovirus is also known as Fifth disease, slapped cheek syndrome, erythema infectiosum. Pathogenic in humans as Parvovirus B-19, it is very common. The incubation period is 13–20 days; it is infectious 10 days before the appearance of a rash and affects around 1 in 400 pregnancies. If suspected in pregnancy, do serology to confirm, and refer to hospital for serial scans to check for hydrops. (Fetal bone marrow suppression causes fetal anaemia, hydrops and death if untreated. Treat with intrauterine transfusion.) CTG shows a sinusoidal baseline in fetal anaemia. Risk to fetus is highest between 4 and 20 weeks gestation.

28 F, T, T, F, T
A good web site is www.chorio.group.shef.ac.uk

29 F, T, T, F, F
One in five deliveries in the UK was induced in 2004–05.
   National Institute for Health and Clinical Excellence. *Induction of Labour: NICE guideline 70.* London: NIHCE; 2008. www.nice.org.uk/guidance/CG070
   Twenty-four hours after pre-labour rupture of membranes at term, induction is advised to be carried out as the risk of sepsis/chorioamnionitis is increased. If macrosomia is simply suspected, it is not an indication for induction of labour. Maternal request is not usually an indication, but special circumstances may necessitate induction. IUD is best managed by induction. If delivery is indicated, IOL can be offered to women with a previous history of Caesarean section. They must be counselled regarding increased risk of uterine rupture and delivery by Caesarean section.

30 T, F, T, T, T
Basal body temperature shows a rise of 0.5°C indicating ovulation has occurred due to the effects of progesterone.

Clear Blue® and First Response® detect LH surge normally 24–36h before ovulation.

Baby Start Focus® uses a microscope to detect fern-like pattern in saliva indicating peak fertility.

Baby Start Male Fertility Test® is a home screening test for low sperm count in men claiming to be 97% accurate in 15 minutes.

Bio-check Fertility® detects FSH levels in urine to determine whether they are rising and as such demonstrating a reduced ability to conceive.

31 T, F, F, T, T
Patients may suffer from clonus and epigastric pains.

32 F, T, F, T, T
Risk factors include: POP because it delays ovum transport (not COCP), increasing age, non-Caucasian race, previous tubal surgery, previous ectopic pregnancy, previous induced abortion, diethylstilboestrol exposure, infertility treatment (e.g. induction of ovulation) and IVF.

Right sided ectopic is thought to be more common than left; this is thought to be due to spread of infection from appendicitis. Depo-provera® and subdermal implant contraception are not risk factors.

33 F, T, F, F, T
There is no benefit of routine ante-natal screening for GBS as there is no obvious benefit in treating GBS carriage ante-natally. However, it is important to consider the intrapartum use of penicillin. The RCOG green-top guideline for GBS advises that it should be 'considered', but most hospitals routinely use intrapartum antibiotics for women with GBS in this pregnancy or who have a history of past GBS carriage. EOGBSD tends to occur in the first seven days of life, occurs by vertical transmission and is more common than late onset. It usually manifests as septicaemia or pneumonia. Late onset can occur up to day 90.

Royal College of Obstetricians and Gynaecologists. *Prevention of Early Onset Neonatal Group B Streptococcal Disease: green-top 36.* London: Royal College of Obstetricians and Gynaecologists; 2003.
www.rcog.org.uk/files/rcog-corp/uploaded-files/GT36GroupB Strep2003.pdf

34 T, F, T, T, T

In one method of diagnosis, three of the four Amsel's criteria must be present: typical discharge, clue cells on wet slide, pH of vaginal discharge >4.5 and release of fishy odour on adding alkali (whiff test). BV is not itchy; discharge is offensive, watery and does not cause soreness. Over 50% of sufferers are asymptomatic. Very common with high rates of recurrence. Treat with oral or vaginal metronidazole/ clindamycin, avoid douching. Treat if symptomatic in pregnancy.
www.bashh.org.uk

35 F, F, F, T, F

National HPV screening started in September 2008 and is offered to all girls aged 12–13 years. Three doses at zero, one and six months complete immunisation. Cervical screening should still be undertaken in vaccinated women as protection is not offered against all subtypes. A two-year catch-up campaign has started in 2009 for girls aged up to 18 years.
www.immunisation.nhs.uk

36 F, T, F, F, T

Hospital care should be delivered for a minimum of 24 hours prior to transfer for community care. It is recommended that a baby is fed as soon as possible post-delivery and preferably within the first 30 minutes. The baby should be fed frequently, approximately every two to three hours until the pre-feed blood sugar is maintained ≥2 mmol/L. Blood glucose should be measured routinely at two to four hours after birth unless indicated earlier.

37 F, F, T, T, F

Turner's is a chromosomal abnormality in girls with the lack of a sex chromosome (XO). Girls tend to have short stature, wide carrying-angles, webbed necks, inverted nipples, broad chests, streak ovaries, coarctation of the aorta and left heart defects.

38 F, T, F, F, T

Capillary haemangiomas (stork marks/salmon patches) are present at birth. They are pale pink patches produced by defects of the dermal capillaries. They are common on the nape and fade with time. Port-wine stains are larger, darker and grow in size. If they are in the distribution of the trigeminal nerve, they may be associated with the neurological condition, Sturge-Weber syndrome. Cavernous haemangiomas (strawberry naevae) are bright red. They occur after birth, increase rapidly in size and then fade by about nine months.

39 T, F, T, T, T

Wilson and Jungner criteria for screening:

- The condition sought should be an important health problem
- There should be an accepted treatment for patients with recognised disease
- Facilities for diagnosis and treatment should be available
- There should be a recognised latent or early symptomatic stage
- There should be a suitable test or examination
- The test should be acceptable to the population
- The natural history of the condition, including development from latent to declared disease, should be adequately understood
- There should be an agreed policy on whom to treat as patients
- The cost of case finding (including diagnosis and treatment of patients diagnosed) should be economically balanced in relation to possible expenditure on medical care as a whole
- Case finding should be a continuous process and not a 'once and for all' project
- Does not say method used for selecting those to be screened should be reliable, only cost effective

Wilson JMG, Jungner G. *Principles and Practice of Screening for Disease.* Geneva: World Health Organization; 1968.

40 T, T, F, F, F

If there is a family history then it is usually linked with the haplotypes HLA-B8 and HLA-Bw16. The patient may present with generalised itching, but more on the palms and soles. There may be jaundice, epigastric discomfort, malaise and excessive bruising/bleeding. Bile salts and liver function tests (LFTs) can all be raised, however, LFTs are rarely higher than three times the normal limits. Ursodeoxycholic acid is not licensed in pregnancy, but many departments use it as it decreases the quantity of bile salts and thus the amount of itching is also reduced. It is essential for the patients to be referred on to a specialist unit to closely monitor fetal wellbeing. Early delivery may be indicated. Oestrogen-dependent contraceptives should be avoided after cholestasis.

Examination B
PAPER 1

EXTENDED MATCHING QUESTIONS

   a   Five days post-natal prophylactic low molecular weight heparin or mechanical methods

   b   Six weeks post-natal prophylactic low molecular weight heparin +/- ante-natal aspirin

   c   Ante-natal and six weeks post-natal prophylactic dose low molecular weight heparin

   d   Hydration and early mobilisation

   e   Ante-natal and six weeks post-natal warfarin

   f   Six weeks post-natal compression stockings and low molecular weight heparin

   g   Low molecular weight heparin and compression stockings until the fifth postoperative day.

For each of the following clinical scenarios relating to thromboprophylaxis, from the list above choose a management option, as recommended by the Royal College of Obstetricians and Gynaecologists. Each option may be used once, more than once or not at all.

   1   A 32-year-old woman with a previous history of DVT on the oral contraceptive pill is pregnant. She has no proven thrombophilia.

   2   A 35-year-old woman with prothrombin gene defect is pregnant. She has no past history of venous thromboembolism.

3 A 30-year-old primiparous woman is undergoing delivery by emergency Caesarean section for failure to progress.

4 A 25-year-old primiparous woman is undergoing delivery by planned Caesarean section for breech presentation.

5 A 32-year-old woman is undergoing a planned delivery by Caesarean section because of a previous Caesarean section. Her mother suffered a DVT.

a Missed abortion

b Septic abortion

c Incomplete miscarriage

d Inevitable miscarriage

e Threatened miscarriage

f Complete miscarriage

g Cervical incompetence

h Antepartum haemorrhage

i Ectopic pregnancy

Concerning types of abortion/miscarriage match the following clinical scenarios. Each type may be used once, more than once or not at all.

6 A 25-year-old lady has had an uneventful pregnancy so far; she is 13 weeks pregnant. However a transvaginal ultrasound demonstrates a fetus of 9 weeks gestation with no cardiac activity.

7 A 30-year-old lady presents with vaginal spotting. She is 25 weeks pregnant and a transvaginal ultrasound demonstrates normal fetal activity.

8 A 40-year-old lady presents at 16 weeks gestation; she is noted to have cervical dilatation of 2 cm and denies any pain or bleeding. She has a past history of dilatation and curettage (D+C) for an incomplete miscarriage at 8 weeks and she has also had a cone biopsy.

9 A 32-year-old lady who is 12 weeks pregnant presents with crampy lower abdominal pain and bleeding. She states she passed a 'large lump of tissue' earlier in the day. On examination her cervix is open.

10 A 26-year-old lady who is 6 weeks pregnant presents with a short history of lower abdominal pain that has now resolved and some vaginal spotting. You have carried out two ßhCG tests 48 hours apart demonstrating a doubling in levels.

    a Monozygotic monochorionic monoamniotic

    b Monozygotic monochorionic diamniotic

    c Dizygotic diamniotic

    d Monozygotic dichorionic diamniotic

    e Conjoined twins

Match the following statements to the correct type of twin pregnancy listed above. Each type may be used once, more than once or not at all.

11 More common in the Nigerian race

12 Has a strong family history

13 More commonly results in cord entanglement

14 Has the highest mortality rate

15 Associated with 'stuck on syndrome'

    a Semen analysis

    b Serum LH:FSH

    c Thyroid function test

    d Diagnostic laparoscopy

    e Tubal patency test

    f Post-coital test

    g Pregnancy test

For the following scenarios, which of the above is the most appropriate test to carry out? Each type may be used once, more than once or not at all.

16 A couple wish to fall pregnant. Neither has had children previously. The woman has a regular menstrual cycle and the man has had an orchidopexy in the past.

17 A couple wish to fall pregnant. The man has had children in the past. The woman had a TOP at age 20 and is otherwise well.

18 A couple wish to fall pregnant. The man has had children in the past. The woman has a BMI of 35 and acne. She has irregular periods.

19 A couple are trying for children. The woman has had normal periods until two years ago. She now complains of severe pain for up to five days before her periods and can pass blood via her back passage during her period.

20 An 18-year-old woman has recently married her childhood sweetheart. They are keen to get pregnant. The woman has noted that for the past two months her periods have become much lighter and her breasts are tender.

a Reassure, no smear test needed

b Smear in five years

c Retest in six months

d Refer for colposcopy

e Smear in three years

f Retest in three months

g Refer for hysterectomy

For each of the following scenarios relating to cervical screening, choose one management option from the list above. Each option may be used once, more than once or not at all.

21 A 53-year-old woman receives a negative result for her smear test.

22 A 35-year-old woman receives a borderline result for her smear test.

23 A 64-year-old woman receives her third consecutive negative result for her smear test.

24 A 48-year-old woman receives an inadequate result for her smear test.

25 A 42-year-old woman receives a second borderline change in squamous cells result for her smear test.

26 A 27-year-old woman receives a negative result for her smear test.

a Post-natal depression

b Generalised anxiety disorder

c Anorexia nervosa

d Depression

e Baby blues

f Schizo-affective disorder

g Puerperal psychosis

h Personality disorder

i Bipolar disorder

For each puerperal psychiatric scenario, choose the most appropriate diagnosis from the above list. Each type may be used once, more than once or not at all.

27 A 27-year-old woman has given birth two weeks ago to a healthy boy. She is feeling tearful when her partner is leaving to go to work in the mornings. She feels tired most of the time. The baby is thriving.

28 A 40-year-old woman has given birth to a child with Down's syndrome two days ago. She does not touch the baby. Her partner is concerned as she does not sleep or eat. She claims that the baby is the devil.

29 A 30-year-old woman, who is known to have a problem with depression in the past, has given birth to a healthy baby girl. She had an extensive perineal tear. Since the delivery she has been on the internet buying clothes for the baby. In a week she has spent over a £1000.

30 A 15-year-old girl has given birth to a healthy baby girl. She is due to go back to school in six months. She has taken to eating small amounts and her mother is concerned about her poor concentration. She is looking after the baby well and the baby is thriving.

SINGLE BEST ANSWER: FOR EACH QUESTION CHOOSE ONE ANSWER ONLY

1 The leading cause of direct maternal death in the first trimester in industrialised countries is:

  a Miscarriage

  b Ectopic pregnancy

  c Infection

  d Pulmonary embolism

  e TOP

2 With respect to the treatment of endometriosis, which one of the following is useful for both dysmenorrhoea and infertility?

  a Medroxyprogesterone acetate 10 mg three times a day for 90 days

  b Tri-cycling the combined oral contraceptive pill

  c Danazol

  d Gonadotropin releasing hormone (GnRH) analogues

  e Laser ablation

3 What level of maximum alcohol consumption during pregnancy is recommended in the Ante-natal Care NICE guidelines 2008?

  a 1–2 units per week during pregnancy

  b 1–2 units per day during pregnancy

  c 1–2 units per day during the second and third trimester

  d 1–2 units per week during the first and second trimester

  e 1–2 units per week during the second and third trimester

4 The most common area of implantation for ectopic pregnancy is:

  a Isthmus of the fallopian tube

  b Fimbria of fallopian tube

  c Abdominal cavity

  d Ampulla of fallopian tube

  e On the ovary

5 Concerning physiological changes in pregnancy, which one of the following is true?

a Human placental lactogen acts as an insulin agonist raising blood sugars and so requiring more insulin, sometimes exposing previous latent diabetes.

b Average weight gain is 28 kilos, with the majority in later half of the pregnancy.

c Haemoglobin levels fall due to iron deficiency.

d Cardiac output increases, but due to a decrease in peripheral resistance blood pressure in normal pregnancy does not rise.

e Iron supplements should be offered to all pregnant women.

6 With reference to the June 2005 NICE guidelines on referral for suspected cancer, which ONE of the following statements is NOT true?

a A previous negative smear test in women with findings suspicious of cervical cancer should not delay referral.

b A cervical smear test is not required before referral in women with findings suspicious of cervical cancer.

c If a woman on HRT presents with persistent postmenopausal bleeding after HRT has been stopped for six weeks, an urgent referral should be made.

d An unexplained palpable pelvic mass should be referred urgently for ultrasound.

e Vulval pain should be referred urgently.

7 According to the October 2006 NICE guidelines for urinary incontinence for suffers of overactive bladder (OAB), what management option should NOT be used routinely?

a Bladder training

b Electrical stimulation

c Intravaginal oestrogens

d Generic oxybutynin

e Tolterodine

8 Risks associated with grand multiparity include all of the following EXCEPT:

  a Uterine atony

  b Pre-eclampsia

  c Amniotic fluid embolism

  d Abnormal lie

  e Stress incontinence

9 Which side effect causes most women to stop using the Implanon® subdermal contraceptive?

  a Acne

  b Weight gain

  c Irregular bleeding

  d Mood disturbances

  e Headaches

10 What is the maximum allowed gestational age for air travel for an uncomplicated pregnancy?

  a 28 weeks

  b 32 weeks

  c 34 weeks

  d 36 weeks

  e 38 weeks

11 In a pregnant woman what value of systolic blood pressure is classified as severe hypertension?

  a $\geq 145\,\text{mmHg}$

  b $\geq 150\,\text{mmHg}$

  c $\geq 160\,\text{mmHg}$

  d $\geq 170\,\text{mmHg}$

  e $\geq 175\,\text{mmHg}$

12 Which ONE of the following is NOT true about continuous combined HRT?

   a Decreases hot flushes

   b Decreases vaginal atrophy

   c Decreases the risk of myocardial infarction

   d Increases the risk of breast cancer

   e Increases the risk of cerebrovascular incidents

13 A 35-year-old woman comes to your surgery complaining of irregular vaginal bleeding. She had a delivery by Caesarean section seven weeks ago. The bleeding is dark and has small clots and is offensive. On examination she is pyrexial, her respiratory rate is 20 breaths per minute; pulse is 90 beats per minute; and her blood pressure is 100/70 mmHg. She is not pale. Her abdomen is tender and the wound is clean and dry. The lochia is offensive. What is the most likely diagnosis?

   a UTI

   b Wound infection

   c Pulmonary embolus

   d Retained products of conception

   e Endometritis

14 What is the accuracy of home pregnancy tests on the first day of a missed period?

   a 60%

   b 80%

   c 90%

   d 95%

   e 97%

15 Which ONE of the following statements is NOT a recommendation by NICE regarding the monitoring of fetal wellbeing and growth in ante-natal care?

   a Measuring the symphysio-fundal height after 24 weeks gestation at each ante-natal appointment is recommended.

   b Routine use of Doppler ultrasound is not recommended in uncomplicated pregnancies.

c   Routine auscultation of the fetal heart is not necessary, but can provide reassurance to the mother.

d   Presentation should be noted prior to 36 weeks.

e   Fetal assessment with CTG in an uncomplicated pregnancy is not recommended.

16 In a pregnant woman with pre-existing diabetes, when should a retinal assessment be recommended?

a   If she has not had a test within the last month

b   If she has not had a test within the last 3 months

c   If she has not had a test within the last 6 months

d   If she has not had a test within the last 9 months

e   If she has not had a test within the last 1 year

17 Causes of second trimester miscarriage include all of the following EXCEPT:

a   Cervical incompetence

b   Bacterial vaginosis

c   Bicornuate uterus

d   Edwards' syndrome

e   Endometriosis

18 A 54-year-old post menopausal woman, who has been on continuous combined HRT for four months, has one episode of vaginal bleeding. What is the best course of management?

a   Refer her under the two-week suspected cancer rule to the hospital.

b   Carry out a full blood count and thyroid function test.

c   Advise her to wait and observe for further bleeding.

d   Change her over to cyclical hormone replacement.

e   Refer her to the gynaecologist as a routine appointment.

Examination B
PAPER 1 ANSWERS

EXTENDED MATCHING QUESTIONS

1 b

2 c

3 a

4 d

5 g

Remember that thromboembolism is a major risk factor for maternal mortality and even a woman undergoing emergency Caesarean section is not low risk. There are risk assessment proformae in the current guidelines and it is worth being familiar with them as women with thrombophilia/previous history of venous thromboembolism will get pregnant and you will have to advise them on possible regimens. Remember to refer for joint obstetrics/haematology ante-natal care. Warfarin is safe post-natally and if breastfeeding.

Royal College of Obstetricians and Gynaecologists. *Report of the RCOG Working Party on Prophylaxis Against Thromboembolism in Gynaecology and Obstetrics*. London: Royal College of Obstetricians and Gynaecologists; 1995.

Royal College of Obstetricians and Gynaecologists. *Thromboprophylaxis During Pregnancy, Labour and After Normal Vaginal Delivery: RCOG guideline no. 37*. London: Royal College of Obstetricians and Gynaecologists; 2004.

6 a

Management is either expectant or with D+C.

7 h

Miscarriage is defined as occurring in pregnancies of <24 weeks gestation.

8 g

An incompetent cervix results in painless cervical dilatation without uterine contractions. Inevitable miscarriage is associated with uterine contraction leading to the cervical dilatation and as such abdominal pain.

9 c

Complications include continued bleeding and risk of infection. Management is D+C.

10 e

Approximately 50% go on to have a miscarriage.

11 c

12 c

13 a

14 e

15 b

Twin pregnancies have a higher risk of complications compared to singleton pregnancies except for postmaturity. Conjoined twins have the highest rate of complications due to the sharing of organs and post delivery surgical requirement. Monozygotic twins have the next highest mortality rate due to twin to twin transfusion. Dizygotic diamniotic twins have the lowest mortality rate. Dizygotic twins have familial and racial preponderance (more common in Nigerians and less common in the Japanese race). Monozygotes have a relatively constant incidence throughout the world and no familial tendency.

16 a

An orchidopexy or infections such as mumps can cause infertility in the male. It is essential to carry out a semen analysis. Multiple specimens may be required. The female in this situation has a regular menstrual cycle and thus is likely to be ovulating regularly.

17 e

In this situation, the male has no obvious problems. However, this woman is experiencing secondary infertility. Of note she has had a termination, which can be complicated with pelvic infections caus-ing tubal patency issues. As she has no other symptoms a diagnostic laparoscopy is not initially indicated.

18 b
This woman may be suffering from PCOS. In this the LH:FSH ratio may be raised. Also, the testosterone level may be increased.

19 d
In this situation the woman may be suffering from endometriosis as characterised by the change in her menstrual cycle and the severity of pain prior to her period. The blood from the back passage may be caused by endometrial deposits in the anal passage.

20 g
This woman is likely to be already pregnant as displayed by her symp-toms. Pregnancy should be considered even though a woman is still having her 'period' especially when the bleeding is lighter or shorter in duration than usual.

21 b

22 c

23 a

24 f

25 c

26 e
Women aged 25 years are invited for their first smear. At age 25–49, smears are repeated every three years. At age 50–64, smears are repeated every five years. At áge 65+, women are only screened if they have not been screened since age 50 or clinically indicated. As this book is being written, the National Screening Programme age ranges are being considered by Parliament. Since the media atten-tion brought by the high profile death of celebrity Jade Goody from cervical carcinoma, campaigners are calling for younger women to be screened.
www.cancerscreening.nhs.uk/cervical

Recall/referral strategies based on test result

Test result	Recommendations for care
Inadequate	Repeat test in three months
	If three consecutive samples are inadequate, refer for colposcopy
Negative	Woman recalled routinely
Borderline nuclear change	Repeat test in six months
	If three tests are reported as borderline change, refer for colposcopy. If three consecutive tests are reported as negative, woman recalled routinely.
Mild dyskaryosis	Minimum standard – if two consecutive tests reported as mild dyskaryosis, refer for colposcopy.
	Best practice – refer for colposcopy after one test reported as mild dyskaryosis.
Moderate dyskaryosis	Immediate referral for colposcopy
Severe dyskaryosis	Immediate referral for colposcopy
Suspected invasive cancer or suspected glandular neoplasia	Urgent referral for colposcopy

These are not comprehensive guidelines, but further information can be obtained from: www.patient.co.uk
www.cancerscreening.nhs.uk/cervical/publications/nhscsp20.html

27 e

Baby blues tend to peak three to four days after delivery and can last up to six weeks. They occur in approximately 50% of women. Features include labile mood, tiredness, tearfulness, and anxiety. Support and education and help with sleep are the best treatment stratagems. NICE advises asking recently delivered mothers about their emotional wellbeing. Remember a diagnosis of post-natal depression can be made if features appear from within the first month to the first year after childbirth. During ante-natal care NICE advises asking mothers screening questions to identify depression.

National Institute for Health and Clinical Excellence. *Routine Post-natal Care of Women and their Babies: NICE guideline 37*. London: NIHCE; 2006. www.nice.org.uk/guidance/CG037

28 g

This lady has paranoid thoughts about her baby. This is puerperal psychosis and tends to occur in women who have had either a difficult pregnancy or delivery. A baby with a disability is another risk factor. Psychosis occurs very soon after delivery and can be life threatening for both the mother and baby. Hence, it is essential to organise quick intervention by the psychiatric services.

29 i

This patient is known to have had problems pre-pregnancy. Her excessive spending post-delivery may be a manifestation of bipolar disorder. It is likely that the pregnancy has triggered a manic stage in this patient's condition.

30 c

This girl is in the typical age group for anorexia nervosa. Even though she has a valid reason for her increased weight, she has a poor self-body image. She is eating less than she should. She has poor concentration due to these factors.

SINGLE BEST ANSWER

1 b

2 e

There is no evidence that medical treatment improves infertility; however, it is useful with symptoms of dysmenorrhoea. Add back HRT reduces loss of bone density when using GnRH analogues. Danazol given for six to nine months produces pseudomenopause, it is a testosterone derivative that suppresses the LH surge, decreases the levels of sex hormone binding globulin, increases free testosterone as well as inhibiting ovarian steroidogenesis, and therefore masculinises the female fetus.

3 e

NICE states there is uncertainty as to the safety limit in pregnancy, but at this level it is unlikely to cause harm to the new born baby. One unit is defined as half a pint of normal strength lager or a small glass of wine.

4 d

Ectopic pregnancy is managed by laparotomy if life threatening. However, laparoscopic salpingectomy or salpingostomy may be performed, depending on the state of the other fallopian tube and if fertility needs to be maintained. Medical treatment includes methotrexate administered intramuscularly, or an intratubal injection into the gestational sac, but it is only used for small early ectopics of <4.0 cm.

5 d
Human placental lactogen is an insulin antagonist not agonist. The average weight gain is 12.5 kg or 28 lb. Haemoglobin levels fall due to haemodilution as plasma volume rises. Women may complain of feeling faint when lying supine during late pregnancy due to vena caval compression by an enlarging uterus. Iron supplements should only be offered to women at high risk of anaemia due to poor nutrition after screening in first trimester and or later in pregnancy if Hb <10 g/dl and mean cell volume (MCV) <84 fl. Other changes include up to a four-fold increase in erythrocyte sedimentation rate (ESR), an increase in white cell count (WCC) due to neutrophilia, an increase in platelets and a decrease in albumin. The cholesterol level also increases in pregnancy as lipids are the main source of energy.

6 e
Vulval pain and pruritis are common symptoms and should initially be managed on a 'treat, watch and wait' policy. However these cases should be followed up and referred if treatment is not successful. An unexplained vulval lump should be referred urgently. If urgent ultrasound services are not available to investigate an unexplained pelvic mass, the woman should be referred urgently to gynaecology.

National Institute for Health and Clinical Excellence. *Referral for Suspected Cancer: NICE guideline 27*. London: NIHCE; 2005. www. nice.org.uk/guidance/CG027

7 b
Bladder training should be used for a minimum of six weeks and if this is ineffective then oxybutynin should be trialled. It is important to warn the patient of the side effects, which can include dry mouth and blurred vision. If oxybutynin is not tolerated then alternatives such as tolterodine and solifenacin can be tried. Intravaginal oestrogen in postmenopausal women can be used routinely. Electrical stimulation is not recommended. Women with a BMI of over 30 should be encouraged to lose weight.

8 b
Grand multiparity is defined as a woman who has delivered four or more infants with a gestational age of 24 weeks or more. Great grand

multiparity is delivery of seven or more infants beyond 24 weeks. Higher risk of pre-eclampsia is associated with primiparity.

9 c

According to the NICE guideline for long-acting reversible contraception, up to 33% of women stop using the Implanon® within the first year due to irregular bleeding. Acne can occur, but there is no evidence of effect on libido, mood, headaches and bone mineral density.

National Institute for Health and Clinical Excellence. *Long-Acting Reversible Contraception: NICE guideline 30.* London: NIHCE; 2005. www.nice.org.uk/guidance/CG030

10 d

Thirty-two weeks for a multiple pregnancy. The mother should contact the airline if she is over 28 weeks' pregnant and have a letter from her doctor stating he/she is happy for her to fly, as well as the mother's gestational age, expected date of delivery and that the patient is in good health. Advise mother to frequently walk, increase water consumption and use air travel elastic compression stockings while flying.

11 d

Systolic blood pressure of ≥170 mmHg and diastolic blood pressure of more than 110 mmHg on two occasions defines severe hypertension. Severe pre-eclampsia is the above with significant proteinuria (>1 g/L in 24 hours).

Royal College of Obstetricians and Gynaecologists. *The Management of Severe Pre-Eclampsia/Eclampsia: green-top 10A.* London: Royal College of Obstetricians and Gynaecologists; 2006. Available at: www. rcog.org.uk/womens-health/clinical-guidance/management-severe-pre-eclampsiaeclampsia-green-top-10a (accessed 16 March 2009).

12 c

It was previously thought that HRT provided a cardioprotective effect. However, newer evidence, provided in part by the Women's Health Initiative Study, has shown that women are at an increased risk of coronary heart disease, especially in the first year after initiating HRT.

www.nhlbi.nih.gov/whi/

13 e

The most likely cause of puerperal sepsis post-Caesarean section is endometritis, not retained products of conception.

National Institute for Health and Clinical Excellence. *Caesarean*

Section: NICE guideline 13. London: NIHCE; 2004. www.nice.org.uk/guidance/CG013

14 c

This article demonstrated that the highest possible screening sensitivity for ßhCG-based pregnancy tests conducted on day one of a missed period is 90%. 10% of fertilised eggs will not have implanted yet and thus will not be producing ßhCG. The authors go on to estimate the sensitivity as 97% one week after the first day of the missed period.

Wilcox A, Day Baird D, Dunson D, *et al.* Natural limits of pregnancy testing in relation to the expected menstrual period. *JAMA.* 2001; **286**(14): 1759–61.

15 d

Noting the presentation of the fetus prior to 36 weeks is not recommended as it may still change. If malpresentation is suspected, ultrasound should always be used to check.

National Institute for Health and Clinical Excellence. *Antenatal Care: Routine care for the healthy pregnant woman: NICE clinical guideline 62.* London: NIHCE; 2008. www.nice.org.uk/guidance/CG055

16 e

This should be a digital assessment with an appropriate mydriatic. If there is any diabetic retinopathy present then a review assessment should be offered at 16–20 weeks. If the previous assessment was normal then a review should be offered at 28 weeks.

National Institute for Health and Clinical Excellence. *Diabetes in Pregnancy: NICE guideline 63.* London: NIHCE; 2008. www.nice.org.uk/guidance/CG063

17 e

Second trimester miscarriages are between 14 and 24 weeks. Uterine abnormalities including fibroids, infections (e.g. parvovirus, CMV and toxoplasmosis) as well as maternal thrombophilia (e.g. antiphospholipid syndrome) are risk factors. Endometriosis is not a cause.

Kortelahti M, Anttila M, Hippeläinen M, *et al.* Obstetric outcome in women with endometriosis: a matched case-control study. *Gynecol Obstet Invest.* 2003; **56**(4): 207–12.

18 c

This scenario does not meet the criteria according to NICE referral for suspected cancer 2005. Most women should be amenorrhoeic on continuous HRT, but for the first six months they may have episodes of vaginal bleeding. This does not warrant an urgent referral. If bleeding occurs after six months or after a time of amennorhoea then endometrial investigations, such as endometrial sampling, are indicated.

The Scottish Intercollegiate Guidelines Network. *Investigation of Postmenopausal Bleeding*. SIGN: Edinburgh; 2002. Available at: www.sign.ac.uk/guidelines/fulltext/61/index.html (accessed 17 March 2009).

Examination B
PAPER 2

MULTIPLE CHOICE QUESTIONS

1 Syphilis:
   a Does not cause ulcers outside of the genital area
   b Secondary syphilis may be latent and asymptomatic for life
   c Can affect bone
   d Is not a cause of stillbirth
   e First line treatment for pregnant women is intramuscular penicillin

2 Rubella in pregnancy:
   a Tends to cause fetal damage if the infection occurs after 16 weeks
   b Immunisation should be given if a pregnant woman is exposed to rubella
   c May cause deafness in the neonate
   d Tends to cause 'salt and pepper' retinopathy in the neonate
   e Causes 'blueberry' skin lesions in the neonate

3 Intrauterine devices.

   a Devices that contain the least amount of copper should be used.

   b Copper coils work primarily by preventing implantation.

   c The Mirena® intrauterine system works primarily by preventing implantation.

   d The highest risk of pelvic infections occurs up to three weeks post-insertion.

   e Copper coils can make the periods longer, heavier and more painful.

4 Which of the following diseases are associated with polyhydramnios?

   a Diabetes mellitus

   b Duodenal atresia

   c Twin-to-twin transfusion syndrome

   d Maternal hypothyroidism

   e Renal agenesis

5 The following are examples of chromosomal abnormalities:

   a Down's syndrome

   b Patau's syndrome

   c Kleinfelter's syndrome

   d Hereditary spherocytosis

   e Congenital adrenal hyperplasia (CAH)

6 Concerning Rhesus disease in pregnancy.

   a This requires a Rhesus positive father and a Rhesus negative mother.

   b Primary exposure can occur with amniocentesis.

   c During primary exposure there is significant haemolysis resulting in anaemia and multi-organ failure.

   d An indirect Coombs test should be performed at the first ante-natal visit in all Rhesus negative mothers.

   e Anti-D immunoglobulin prophylaxis should be given to all Rhesus negative women not sensitised soon after delivery.

7 A normal sperm analysis includes the following:

a Volume >2 mL

b Motility >30%

c Normal forms >50%

d Concentration >20 × 10⁶/mL

e Red cells <5 × 10⁹

8 Placental types associated with post-partum haemorrhage include:

a Placenta praevia

b Placenta increta

c Succenturiate lobe

d Placenta membranacea

e Battledore placenta

9 Uterovaginal prolapse.

a Prolapse of the posterior vaginal wall is known as a cystocele.

b A second degree uterine prolapse is one in which the cervix reaches the introitus.

c An enterocele may present with a small bowel obstruction.

d A ring pessary can be used as a conservative treatment and needs to be inserted into the anterior fornix.

e HRT is a widely-used conservative treatment option.

10 With regards to malaria prophylaxis in pregnancy.

a Chemoprophylaxis is 100% protective.

b Malaria should be considered if a patient presents with a febrile illness one week to one year after entering a malaria area.

c Malaria is transmitted by the Anopheles mosquito.

d Chloroquine has not be shown to have adverse effects.

e DEET is contraindicated.

11 Risk factors for endometrial cancer include:
   a COCP
   b Obesity
   c PCOS
   d Diabetes mellitus
   e Late menopause

12 Concerning the normal stages of labour.
   a Pushing should start in the active phase of the first stage of labour.
   b Water births have a shorter first stage of labour.
   c The cervix dilates at 1 cm per hour at the start of labour.
   d Expectant management is preferred to active management in the third stage of labour.
   e Ergometrine is associated with hypertension.

13 Fibroids may undergo the following changes:
   a Hyaline change
   b Cystic change
   c Infection
   d Torsion
   e Calcification

14 The Apgar system is made of the following variables:
   a Muscle tone
   b Respiratory effort
   c Heart rate
   d Reflex/irritability
   e Colour

15 Anxiety is reduced at colposcopy by:
   a Listening to music during the procedure
   b Providing information leaflets
   c Playing information videos about colposcopy prior to the procedure

   d Viewing a video of the colposcopy taking place

   e Having a doctor rather than a nurse colposcopist

16 Essential blood tests in the management of pre-eclampsia are:

   a Full blood count (FBC)

   b Thyroid function tests

   c Renal function

   d Liver function

   e Clotting studies

17 Vulval ulceration is commonly caused by the following:

   a Behçet's disease

   b Syphilis

   c Herpes

   d Vulval cancer

   e Diabetes mellitus

18 Breastfeeding.

   a Suckling stimulates the anterior pituitary gland to produce oxytocin, which is important in milk secretion.

   b Suckling stimulates the posterior pituitary gland to produce prolactin, which is important in the 'let down' of milk.

   c Breast cancer is less likely the longer a woman breast feeds her baby.

   d Breast-fed babies have less chance of developing type 1 diabetes mellitus.

   e Bromocriptine can be used to inhibit lactation by inhibiting oxytocin release.

19 TOP increases the risk of:

   a Subsequent infertility

   b Future placenta praevia

   c Future miscarriage

   d Future preterm delivery

   e Future breast cancer

20 Alcohol in pregnancy.

   a Alcohol is the commonest teratogen.

   b Developmental delay is a feature of fetal alcohol syndrome.

   c The Department of Health advises to avoid consumption completely.

   d Binge drinking in pregnancy is especially risky.

   e Fetal alcohol syndrome (FAS) incidence is around 0.6 per 1000 live births.

21 Post coital bleeding (PCB) is a symptom in the following conditions:

   a *Trichomonas vaginalis* infection

   b Cervical ectropion

   c *Chlamydia pecorum* infection

   d Cervical polyp

   e Bacterial vaginosis infection

22 Breech presentation:

   a Incidence is approximately 6% at term

   b 85% of breech presentations are frank breech

   c Is associated with higher rates of perinatal mortality regardless of mode of delivery

   d Should be suspected if the fetal heart can be heard loudest above the maternal umbilicus at 24 weeks

   e Is associated with congenital dysplasia of the hip

23 Regarding benign ovarian tumours.

   a CA-125 is of no benefit.

   b Mucinous cystadenomas can contain well differentiated material (e.g. hair and teeth).

   c Benign germ cell tumours are most common in young women.

   d Hypothyroidism is a risk factor.

   e They can present with ascites.

24 The following factors reduce the likelihood of Caesarean section:

   a Epidural analgesia

   b Immersion in water during labour

   c Continuous intrapartum support from a female

   d Partogram with four-hour action line

   e Drinking raspberry leaf tea

25 Concerning PCOS.

   a One-third of females in the UK suffer from PCOS.

   b Over 50% of PCOS sufferers have raised testosterone levels.

   c PCOS sufferers have an increased risk of transient ischaemic attacks (TIA) and strokes.

   d PCOS sufferers should be screened for ovarian cancer as the incidence is higher.

   e A proposed theory involves insulin resistance in adipose tissue and skeletal muscle with insulin sensitivity of the ovary.

26 Fetal CTG.

   a This is recommended to be used with all women in labour.

   b The rate of operative intervention due to fetal distress is significantly decreased when both fetal CTG and PR-interval analysis is used in labour.

   c Using both fetal CTG and PR-interval analysis during labour significantly improves neonatal outcome.

   d Routine use has increased rates of operative and instrumental delivery.

   e An acceleration is defined as a rise from the baseline of 10 beats per minute lasting for 10 seconds.

27 Regarding dysmenorrhoea.

    a Non-steroidal anti-inflammatory drugs (NSAIDs) are an effective treatment in 80–90% of cases.

    b Coils lead to worsening dysmenorrhoea except the Mirena®, which may be beneficial.

    c Secondary dysmenorrhoea is uncommon before 25 years of age.

    d The COCP is a useful treatment for primary dysmenorrhoea.

    e The pain in secondary dysmenorrhoea is constant throughout the period whilst in primary dysmenorrhoea peaks during the first two days.

28 Cord prolapse is associated with the following:

    a Breech delivery

    b Polyhydramnios

    c Multiparity

    d Macrosomia

    e Male fetus

29 Hydatidiform mole.

    a This can present with hyperemesis gravidarum.

    b ßhCG should be monitored for two years after treatment.

    c It is less common in mothers <20 years and also >40 years.

    d Complete hydatidiform moles are always 46XX karyotype.

    e The combined oral contraceptive can be started one month after ßhCG is undetectable.

30 Perineal trauma.

    a This is common during vaginal delivery.

    b A third degree perineal tear involves the perineal deep musculature and vagina only.

    c A fourth degree perineal tear involves the anal epithelium.

    d It is more common after the first delivery.

    e May be anterior or posterior.

31 Tests for antiphospholipid syndrome include:

   a Dilute Russell viper venom time

   b Anticardiolipin antibody IgG

   c Antiphospholipid antibody profile

   d Activated partial thromboplastin time

   e Anticardiolipin antibody IgM

32 Stillbirth.

   a This is classified as a perinatal death by the Office for National Statistics.

   b This is defined by law as any 'child' expelled or issued forth by its mother after the 20th week of pregnancy that did not breathe or show any other signs of life.

   c Registration is entered into the standard Register of Births.

   d Registration is optional.

   e A Certificate of Stillbirth is issued with documentation for cremation or burial.

33 Beneficial for the treatment of cyclical mastalgia:

   a Topical NSAIDs

   b Pyridoxine

   c Progestogens

   d Evening primrose oil

   e GnRH analogues

34 Epilepsy in pregnancy.

   a The risk of a child inheriting epilepsy from its mother is around 1% for most types of epilepsy.

   b Around 40–50% of epileptic women will experience an increase in seizure frequency.

   c Around 0.5% of women attending ante-natal clinics in the UK are taking antiepileptic drugs.

   d Around 4% of maternal deaths were due to epilepsy according to the most recent Confidential Enquiry into Maternal and Child Health (CEMACH).

   e Carbamazepine causes more major fetal anomalies than valproate.

35 Concerning chorionic villus sampling (CVS).

    a It is usually performed between 10 and 13 weeks gestation.

    b It is usually carried out via the trans-abdominal approach.

    c It can be used to detect neural tube defects.

    d The background pregnancy loss is approximately 2%.

    e It is more accurate in diagnosis than amniocentesis.

36 For pregnant women, which of the following infections are screened for at booking?

    a Chlamydia

    b Hepatitis B

    c Hepatitis C

    d CMV

    e Syphilis

37 Emergency contraception.

    a It needs to be taken within 36 hours.

    b The sooner the patient takes the tablet the more effective it is.

    c If a patient has a large bout of diarrhoea or vomits within three hours of the tablet being taken, they must take another tablet.

    d The Mirena® coil can be effective if used within five days of unprotected sexual intercourse (UPSI).

    e The copper coil may be used up to day 19 of a 28-day cycle.

38 Regarding operative (instrumental, assisted) vaginal delivery.

    a The rate of achieving a normal vaginal delivery after operative delivery is 80%.

    b Prophylactic antibiotics are indicated for operative delivery.

    c Ventouse extraction is more likely to be associated with failure of delivery than forceps delivery.

    d Ventouse extraction is less likely to be associated with maternal worries about the baby.

    e Forceps delivery is more likely to be associated with low five-minute Apgar scores than ventouse extraction.

39 Congenital adrenal hyperplasia.
  a It is due to 21-hydroxylase deficiency.
  b Sufferers have ambiguous genitalia.
  c It can cause vomiting and dehydration.
  d Some babies are genetically identified as male.
  e It may cause infertility later in life.

40 Causes of respiratory distress in a newborn:
  a Infection
  b Meconium aspiration
  c Intrapartum asphyxia
  d Hypothyroidism
  e Myasthenia gravis

Examination B
PAPER 2 ANSWERS

MULTIPLE CHOICE

1   F, T, T, F, T

Syphilis is caused by the spirochaete *Treponema pallidum* and is becoming more common. It can be transmitted sexually, via contact with an infectious lesion, or via contaminated blood products or vertical transmission can occur during pregnancy. It is classified as congenital or acquired, early (primary, secondary or early latent within two years of infection) or late (tertiary or late latent after two years of infection). Diagnosis is usually serological but *T. pallidum* can be visualised under dark ground microscopy from, for example, ulcer scrapings. It is associated with HIV infection. Primary syphilis presents with a solitary painless ulcer and painless lymphadenopathy most commonly, **but** can present with pain as well. Secondary syphilis is characterised by systemic symptoms: fever, malaise, aches and pains, typical rash and condylomata lata. If early syphilis is left untreated, vertical transmission rates can be as high as 70–100% with up to one-third resulting in stillbirth. Latent syphilis is characterised by positive serology in the absence of symptoms/signs. Tertiary syphilis clinically presents with involvement in three areas: cardiovascular, neurological, and gummata – nodules/plaques that have a preponderance for bone and skin. Treatment is with intramuscular penicillin.

Kingston M, French P, Goh B, *et al.* UK national guidelines on the management of syphilis 2008. *Int J STD AIDS.* 2008; **19**(11): 729–40.

2   F, F, T, T, T

If rubella occurs in the mother up to the first 8–10 weeks of gestation, there is a 90% chance of damage to the fetus. This declines to 10–20% risk of damage by 16 weeks and after this time damage to the fetus is rare. Congenital rubella syndrome can cause deafness, retinopathy and skin lesions, which can be purpuric ('blueberry lesions'). Cataracts, mental retardation and heart defects are also common. Immunisation is contraindicated in pregnancy and pregnancy should be avoided for three months post-vaccination.

3   F, T, T, T, T
Copper coils should use at least 300 mm² of copper; currently the most common IUD in usage has 380 mm². IUDs work by preventing implantation and also by the copper, which makes the cervical mucus inhospitable to sperm. The IUS works by preventing implantation and occasionally by preventing fertilisation. The IUD can make the periods more heavy and painful; that is one of the main reasons women have the IUD removed. The IUS is licensed for heavy menstrual bleeding as it tends to make periods lighter and shorter in duration. However, initially the IUS can make periods more irregular. Coil checks should be undertaken after three to six weeks.

National Institute for Health and Clinical Excellence. *Long-Acting Reversible Contraception: NICE guideline 30*. London: NIHCE; 2005. www.nice.org.uk/guidance/CG030

4   T, T, T, F, F
Polyhydramnios is a total fluid volume of 2000 mL or more. A quantitative approach of assessment is termed the amniotic fluid index (AFI): using ultrasound, the uterine cavity is split into four quadrants, with the largest pocket being measured in each quadrant and then totalled together and compared to a standardised graph. Polyhydramnios is diagnosed when the AFI is more than the 95th percentile, with normal values available from 16 weeks of gestation. Normally, fetal swallowing causes a reduction in the fluid volume. An absence of swallowing or blockage of the fetal gastrointestinal tract (GIT) may lead to polyhydramnios and therefore is strongly linked to fetal abnormality. Other causes include: oesophageal atresia, muscular dystrophy, severe fetal anaemia, congenital syphilis, placental arterio-venous fistula, placental angioma, viral hepatitis, maternal substance abuse, chromosomal abnormalities (e.g. Down's syndrome), gastrochisis and anencephaly. Fetal hypothyroidism may cause polyhydramnios if goitre is large enough to block swallowing of amniotic fluid. Complications include higher risk of low Apgar scores, low birth weight, preterm labour, Caesarean section, placental abruption, malpresentation, post-partum haemorrhage and cord prolapse.

IM steroids should be given ante-natally if preterm delivery is considered, to improve lung maturity.

5 T, T, T, F, F
Down's syndrome is due to trisomy of chromosome 21. Patau's syndrome is due to trisomy of chromosome 13 and Kleinfelter's syndrome is characteristically displayed as XXY. Hereditary spherocytosis is an example of an inborn error of metabolism. CAH is usually caused by recessive gene defects of steroidogenesis.

6 T, T, F, T, F
The maternal immune system is stimulated to produce antibodies, during primary exposure of Rhesus antigen by fetal maternal blood transfer. There are rarely problems during this exposure, however subsequent pregnancies result in the production of large amounts of maternal anti-D antibodies which can cross the placenta, binding to the fetal red cells and being recognised as foreign by the immune system of the fetus. These red cells are then haemolysed by fetal macrophages and lymphocytes. Anti-D antibodies are not required if both parents are Rhesus negative.

Anti-D immunoglobulin is also given to affected females at other sensitising events, such as abortion, miscarriage, amniocentesis, CVS, cordocentesis, ectopic pregnancy and abdominal trauma. It is also given routinely at 28 and 34 weeks of pregnancy.

7 T, F, F, T, F
The red cell number is not included in sperm analysis. Motility should be more than 50% and normal morphology should be above 30%.

8 T, T, T, T, F
Placenta accreta is a morbid adherence of the placenta to the uterus; however it does not penetrate the myometrium. Placenta increta is a deeper penetration of the placenta into the myometrium. Placenta percreta is the term associated with the placenta crossing the uterine wall into the peritoneum; it may also attach to other organs (e.g. bowel or bladder). Risk factors for placenta accreta/increta and percreta include previous Caesarean section, placenta praevia and advanced maternal age. Battledore placenta is of no clinical significance and is the term used when the cord has a marginal rather than central insertion.

9 F, T, T, F, F
A prolapse of the posterior vaginal wall is a rectocele and a cystocele

is a prolapse of the anterior vaginal wall and bladder. Prolapse of the urethra is known as a urethrocele. A first degree prolapse is one in which there is cervical descent, but it does not reach the introitus. A third degree prolapse is one in which the cervix and uterine body lies outside of the introitus (procidentia). Enteroceles may present with bowel obstruction, but this is rare and is caused by incarceration. A ring pessary needs to be inserted to occupy the posterior fornix and the lower part of anterior vaginal wall. It should be changed at least every six months. If it is incorrectly fitted it can cause a great deal of discomfort and erosions. A ring pessary is effective for anterior vaginal and uterovaginal prolapses. HRT, in any form, will only help with some of the symptoms associated with a prolapse (e.g. vaginal dryness/irritation). It is not a widely-used treatment option as surgery is the mainstay.

10 F, T, T, T, F

No chemoprophylaxis is 100% protective therefore high risk patients (e.g. pregnant women, infants), should avoid travel to malaria zones. Chloroquine and proguanil are the preferred chemoprophylaxis drugs in the first trimester. Mefloquine can be given in the second and third trimester. DEET is safe in pregnancy.

Koren G, Matsui D, Bailey B. DEET-based insect repellents: safety implications for children and pregnant and lactating women. *CMAJ*. 2003; **169**(3): 209–12. Available at: www.cmaj.ca/cgi/content/full/169/3/209 (accessed 17 March 2009).

Pregnancy should be avoided for one week after doxycycline use and three months after mefloquine. Doxycycline is contraindicated in pregnancy as adverse affects include discolouration and dysplasia of teeth as well as inhibition of bone growth.

www.malariasite.com

11 F, T, T, T, T

The COCP (combined oral contraceptive pill) is protective.

12 F, T, F, F, T

First stage starts with contractions and is divided into two phases: (i) latent with effacement and dilatation of the cervix to 3–4 cm; and (ii) active, which leads to full dilatation (10 cm) usually at a rate of 1 cm/hr. The second stage leads on from the first and finishes with delivery of the baby. Women should start pushing with contractions at this stage. The woman should adopt her most comfortable position during this phase. The third stage is from birth of the baby to delivery of the placenta and membranes. Syntometrine (ergometrine and oxytocin) is superior at decreasing PPH than oxytocin alone; however, there is increased incidence of nausea, vomiting and hypertension. Water births have also been associated with a lower rate of episiotomy and analgesic requirements.

13 T, T, T, T, T
Hyaline change may occur when the blood supply slowly diminishes. Liquefaction of the areas of hyaline results in cysts. After curettage, delivery or abortion, for example, a subendometrial fibroid may become infected. A pedunculated fibroid can undergo torsion. Fibroids in postmenopausal women can calcify.

14 T, T, T, T, T
The Apgar system was devised in 1953 by Dr Virginia Apgar. It is measured at one and five minutes post delivery and scores of 0, 1 or 2 are allotted.

	0	1	2
Heart rate	Absent	<100/min	>100/min
Respiratory effort	Absent	Irregular, shallow, weak	Regular, crying well
Reflex/irritability	None	Grimace	Cough/cry
Muscle tone	Limp	Some flexion	Active, well flexed
Colour	Blue/pale	Blue extremities and pink body	Pink

15 T, F, T, T, F
Leaflets did not decrease anxiety, but did increase knowledge. There is no evidence to suggest nurse/doctor colposcopist differences.

Galaal K, Deane K, Sangal S, *et al*. Interventions for reducing anxiety in women undergoing colposcopy. *Cochrane Database Syst Rev.* 2007; **3**: CD006013.

16 T, F, T, T, F
In order to monitor for HELLP syndrome (haemolysis, elevated liver function tests, low platelets) the FBC and LFTs are necessary. However, clotting tests are not routinely needed unless the platelet count drops below 100×10^6/l. Thyroid function tests are not indicated.

Royal College of Obstetricians and Gynaecologists. *Management of Severe Eclampsia/Pre-Eclampsia: RCOG guideline no. 10(A)*. London: Royal College of Obstetricians and Gynaecologists; 2006

17 T, T, T, T, F

18 F, F, T, T, F

The anterior pituitary produces prolactin, which is important in milk secretion. The ejection of milk i.e. the 'let down' is stimulated by the production of oxytocin from the posterior pituitary. Breast and ovarian cancer are less likely in women who have had children and the likelihood of breast cancer decreases with increasing duration of breast feeding. Breast milk contains many protective elements such as lysozymes, IgA and lactoferrin. Babies fed on formula milk are more likely to develop necrotising enterocolitis, respiratory infections, ear infections, asthma/eczema and type 1 diabetes mellitus. Firm breast support and not suckling should be enough to suppress lactation; however, to stop it fully bromocriptine can be used as this inhibits prolactin.

Collaborative Group on Hormonal Factors in Breast Cancer. Breast cancer and breast feeding: collaborative reanalysis of individual data from 47 epidemiological studies in 30 countries, including 50 302 women with breast cancer and 96 973 without the disease. *Lancet.* 2002; **360**(9328): 187–95.

19 F, F, T, T, F

www.rcog.org.uk/resources/Public/pdf/abortion_summary.pdf

20 T, T, F, T, T

Department of Health and NICE guidelines limit consumption of alcohol to one or two units once or twice a week and to avoid intoxication. Most studies on lay people's understandings of units have found that they tend to underestimate units in a drink. Full blown FAS incidence is 0.6 per 1000 live births, but fetal alcohol spectrum disorder (FASD), which may have some features of FAS, is much more common with around 9 in 1000 live births in USA.

Royal College of Obstetricians and Gynaecologists. *Alcohol Consumption and the Outcomes of Pregnancy: statement no. 5.* London: Royal College of Obstetricians and Gynaecologists; 2006. Available at: www.rcog.org.uk/womens-health/clinical-guidance/alcohol-consumption-and-outcomes-pregnancy (accessed 19 March 2009).

National Institute for Health and Clinical Excellence. *Ante-natal Care: routine care for the healthy pregnant woman: NICE guideline 62.* London: NIHCE; 2008. www.nice.org.uk/guidance/CG062

21 T, T, F, T, F

PCB is a symptom of *Chlamydia trachomatis*. BV does not cause PCB.

22 F, T, T, F, T

The incidence of breech births is around 3% at term. The most common presentation is frank breech. Higher rates of perinatal mortality may be related to higher rates of fetal/maternal abnormalities. It should be suspected if the heart can be heard loudest above the umbilicus after around 35 weeks. Risk factors for breech presentation include: high parity, maternal diabetes, fetal anomaly, placenta praevia and maternal smoking.

www.patient.co.uk

Rayl J, Gibson PJ, Hickok DE. A population-based case-control study of risk factors for breech presentation. *Am J Obstet Gynecol.* 1996; **174**(1 Pt 1): 28–32.

23 F, F, T, T, T

CA-125 will help to differentiate between benign/malignant tumours. Benign cystic teratomas (dermoid cysts) can contain teeth and hair, bone, cartilage, muscle and even bronchial or alimentary epithelium. These are germ cell tumours and the commonest type. The most common age of presentation is late teens to early thirties and the cysts can be bilateral. Treatment is with cystectomy. Mucinous cystadenomas are the most common large ovarian tumours, which, if left untreated, can grow to fill the abdominal cavity. The cysts contain mucin and if ruptured, may cause pseudomyxoma peritonei. Meigs tumour is benign and can present with ascites.

www.patient.co.uk

24 F, F, T, T, F

Receiving continuous support from a woman, whether trained or untrained, will reduce the likelihood of CS. In addition, morbidity at Caesarean section is reduced by planned Caesarean section after 39 weeks, which is associated with reduced morbidity of fetal respiratory problems, antibiotic prophylaxis and regional anaesthesia. Antacids and antiemetics reduce morbidity of aspiration pneumonia. A group and save/cross-match is not necessary for healthy women with uncomplicated pregnancies undergoing Caesarean section.

National Institute for Health and Clinical Excellence. *Caesarean Section: NICE guideline 13*. London: NIHCE; 2004. www.nice.org.uk/guidance/CG013

25 F, F, T, F, T

One-third of females in the UK have polycystic ovaries (10 or more follicles per ovary); of these, one-third have PCOS (i.e. together with one or more of hirsutism, acne, male pattern baldness, amenorrhoea or oligomenorrhea, raised testosterone [30%] and or luteinizing hormone [40%]). It has been suggested that hyperinsulinaemia leads to increased androgen excretion by the ovaries and inhibits production of sex hormone binding globulin in the liver. PCOS sufferers are more likely to have raised central obesity, high blood pressure, hypertriglyceridemia, as well as a low HDL cholesterol, compared to normal females of their age and therefore are twice as likely to develop diabetes and three times more likely to develop TIA/strokes. There is also an increased risk of infertility and endometrial cancer.

26 F, F, F, T, F

NICE does not recommend the use of CTG routinely in women with an uncomplicated pregnancy. Its specificity and sensitivity have been called into question and in fact adding in PR-interval analysis of the fetus does not decrease operative intervention nor improve neonatal outcome significantly. Routine use has contributed to increasing rates of operative and instrumental delivery. An acceleration is a rise from the baseline of 15 bpm lasting for 15 seconds.

Strachan BK, van Wijngaarden WJ, Sahota D, *et al.*, for the Fetal electrocardiotocography (FECG) Study Group. Cardiotocography only versus cardiotocography plus PR-interval analysis in intrapartum surveillance: a randomised, multicentre trial. *Lancet*. 2000; **355**(9202): 456–9.

27 T, T, T, T, T

NSAIDs are more effective if started one day before menstruation begins. Primary dysmenorrhoea is generally associated with ovulation and has no detectable pathology unlike secondary dysmenorrhoea that has detectable pathology. Primary dysmenorrhoea usually starts a year after menarche with peak incidence between 15 and 25 years of age. Causes of secondary dysmenorrhoea include adenomyosis, endometriosis, PID and fibroids.

28 T T T T T

Cord prolapse has been defined as the descent of the umbilical cord through the cervix alongside (occult) or past the presenting part (overt) in the presence of ruptured membranes. Fetal compromise occurs as the cord is exposed to the cold and undergoes vasospasm. Also, the cord will be compressed during contractions if in labour. Abnormal lie is associated with cord prolapse, breech 10% and transverse lie up to 20%. Cord prolapse is uncommon, with an incidence between 1 and 6/1000 deliveries. It is an obstetric emergency. It may be indicated by variable decelerations on the CTG. The mother should be placed in the knee-chest position, pressure should be placed on the presenting part to move it away from the cord and arrange delivery by emergency Caesarean section as soon as possible.

Royal College of Obstetricians and Gynaecologists. *Umbilical Cord Prolapse: green-top 50*. London: Royal College of Obstetricians and Gynaecologists; 2008.
www.rcog.org.uk/files/rcog-corp/uploaded-files/GT50 UmbilicalCordProlapse2008.pdf

29 T, T, T, F, T
Hydatidiform moles occur in 1 in 2500–5000 pregnancies in the UK. Two per cent of moles are ultimately diagnosed as choriocarcinoma. It can be complete, with absence of fetal vessels, extensive trophoblastic tissue and hydropic villi (ultrasonographically described as 'snow storm' appearance); or incomplete with some fetal vessels and normal villi present. A chest x-ray should exclude pulmonary metastasis. It is more common in Asian and Taiwanese women where the incidence can be as high as 1 in 200. It is 40 times more common in those who have a past history. They are typically 46XX with both X chromosomes derived from the father; however, some are 46XY. Incomplete moles are typically triploid karyotype 80% 69XXY with the remainder 69 XXX or 69 XYY.

30 T, F, T, T, T
Perineal trauma is common, affecting over 85% of women undergoing spontaneous or assisted vaginal delivery. It can be anterior (affecting, e.g. anterior vagina/clitoris/urethra/labia) or posterior (affecting, e.g. posterior vagina, perineal muscles, anal sphincter). A tear is more common in primigravida women. A first degree tear involves the vaginal skin only. A second degree tear extends into the perineal deep muscles. A third degree tear extends into the anal sphincter and a fourth degree tear extends into the anal epithelium.

McCandlish R, Bowler U, van Asten H, *et al*. A randomised controlled trial of care of the perineum during second stage of normal labour. *Br J Obstet Gynaecol*. 1998; **105**(12): 1262–72.

Risk factors for perineal trauma include large fetal size, malpresentation, malposition, maternal ethnicity (white more than black) and older mothers.

31 T, T, F, F, T
The tests need to be positive on two or more occasions six weeks apart to confirm diagnosis. Treatment involves use of low dose aspirin and heparin to reduce placental infarction and thrombosis.

32 T, F, F, F, T
Stillbirth is defined by law as any 'child' expelled or issued forth by its mother after the 24th week of pregnancy that did not breathe or show any other signs of life. The stillbirth must be registered, and is entered into the Stillbirth Register, which is separate from the standard Register of Births. A Certificate of Stillbirth is then issued with documentation for cremation or burial. It is classified as a perinatal death by the Office for National Statistics. Perinatal deaths include stillbirths and early neonatal deaths.
Royal College of Obstetricians and Gynaecologists. *Registration of Stillbirths and Certification of Pregnancy Loss Before 24 Weeks of Gestation: RCOG good practice no. 4.* London: Royal College of Obstetricians and Gynaecologists; 2005. www.rcog.org.uk

33 T, F, F, F, T
Cyclical mastalgia is breast pain, usually of the outer quadrant, associated with increased lumpiness from mid-cycle and relieved with menstruation. The symptoms are unchanged with pregnancy or OCP, but decline with menopause. *BMJ Clinical Evidence* suggests that the only treatment of benefit is topical NSAIDs, with other treatments involving danazol, gesterone, tamoxifen and GnRH analogues being a trade off between benefit and harm.
Bundred N. Breast pain. *Clinical Evidence.* London: BMJ Publishing Group; 2007. www.clinicalevidence.com

34 F, F, T, T, F
The risk of a child inheriting most types of epilepsy from its mother is around 3%, but may be more. Around one-quarter of women experience more seizures in pregnancy. Eleven women out of 295 died from epilepsy in the last CEMACH report – six from sudden unexplained death in epilepsy (SUDEP). Major fetal anomalies are more common with valproate (5.9%) than either carbamazepine or lamotrigine

(2% for both). The Royal Society of Medicine guidelines are very comprehensive and are written especially for GPs.

Epilepsy Guidelines Group. *Primary Care Guidelines for the Management of Females with Epilepsy.* London: The Royal Society of Medicine Press Ltd; 2004.

35 T, T, F, T, F

CVS can also be carried out via a trans-cervical catheter; however, this has a higher rate of pregnancy loss and failed attempts due to maternal cell contaminant. Results from CVS are usually obtained within 7–14 days, allowing earlier diagnosis, and as such, an opportunity for termination if there's a fetal abnormality. Amniocentesis is slightly more accurate than CVS due to placental mosaicism (i.e. the placenta may have different populations of cells with different karyotype/genotype).

36 F, T, F, F, T

HIV and rubella are also tested for. Toxoplasmosis is not.

National Institute for Health and Clinical Excellence. *Ante-natal Care: routine care for the healthy pregnant woman: NICE guideline 62.* London: NIHCE; 2008. www.nice.org.uk/guidance/CG062

37 F, T, T, F, T

Levonorgestrel 150 mg stat is licensed for use up to 72 hours after UPSI, but on discussion with the patient, if a coil were not appropriate, the pill may be used up to 120 hours post UPSI. However, the sooner the tablet is used the more effective. If used within the 72 hours it is 84% effective and 63% after 72 hours. The copper coil is licensed for emergency contraception and is 99% effective within 5 days. The Mirena® coil is not licensed for emergency contraception.

FFPRHC Guidance. Emergency contraception. *Journal of Family Planning and Reproductive Health Care.* 2006; **32**(2): 121–8.

38 T, F, T, F, F

Women should be advised of the high chance of vaginal delivery following operative delivery. Prophylactic antibiotics are not currently advised. In a Cochrane review of ventouse delivery vs forceps, it was found that ventouse deliveries were more likely to fail, be associated with cephalhaematoma, be associated with retinal haemorrhage and be associated with maternal worries about the baby. Ventouse extraction was less likely to be associated with significant maternal perineal/

vaginal trauma and no more likely to be associated with delivery by CS, low 5 minute Apgar scores, or the need for phototherapy.

Johanson RB, Menon V. Vacuum extraction versus forceps for assisted vaginal delivery. *Cochrane Database Syst Rev.* 1999; **2**: CD000224.

39 T, T, T, T, T

In most cases 21-hydroxylase is the deficient enzyme. In the early weeks it can interfere so profoundly with adrenal and cortisol function that salt-wasting may cause significant vomiting and dehydration. Approximately 90% of babies are identified genetically as female and it is imperative to involve specialists at the earliest stage to clarify the situation. In mild cases, the external genitalia may be ambiguous, but the female may have normal internal sexual organs and thus fertility may not be an issue. However, any degree of severity may make infertility a more significant problem.

40 T, T, T, F, T

Infections can be acquired before or during delivery. Meconium is particularly toxic to the delicate airways of a newborn and can cause significant problems. Asphyxia can cause CNS depression which can lead to respiratory problems. Any muscular/intercostal/diaphragmatic problem could cause respiratory distress.

Examination C
PAPER 1

EXTENDED MATCHING QUESTIONS

    a Ruptured corpus luteal cyst

    b Torsion of the ovary

    c Placental abruption

    d Pre-term labour

    e Acute appendicitis

    f Red degeneration

    g Acute pyelonephritis

Match the above causes of abdominal pain in pregnancy with the following scenarios. Each option may be used once, more than once, or not at all.

1 A 30-year-old Afro-Caribbean lady presents at 14 weeks gestation with right lower quadrant abdominal pain and vomiting. She has had one previous miscarriage and was investigated for infertility in the past. She is apyrexial and has a normal pulse and blood pressure. She is very tender in her right iliac fossa, with an ill-defined mass in the region.

2 A 34-year-old female G2 P. 1 is 16 weeks pregnant and presents with a two-day history of colicky left lower abdominal pain, with nausea and vomiting. The pain is intense with guarding on examination.

3 A 28-year-old G3 P. 1+1 presents at 30 weeks gestation with sudden onset of abdominal pain and vaginal bleeding. She is a smoker, but denies drug use. Her blood pressure is 160/90 mmHg and she is tachycardic. She has a hard, tender uterus.

a Retained products of conception

b Genital tract trauma

c Uterine atony

d Uterine inversion

e Placenta accreta

f Endometritis

Concerning post-partum haemorrhage (PPH), match the following scenarios with the likely cause. Each option may be used once, more than once or not at all.

4 A 35-year-old G4 P. 3 woman who has type 1 diabetes mellitus has a spontaneous delivery at 39 weeks. The baby is large for dates and also the pregnancy was complicated with polyhydramnios. Delivery was uneventful; however after the third stage she has brisk vaginal bleeding that is estimated to be over one litre.

5 A 32-year-old G4 P. 2+1 woman has had one normal delivery, one delivery by Caesarean section and an incomplete miscarriage at 10 weeks gestation requiring dilatation and curettage. At 38 weeks an ultrasound scan noted she had continuing minor placenta praevia. Spontaneous vaginal delivery was successful at 39 weeks plus 3 days. The third stage of labour, however, was prolonged with placental delivery not complete after 30 minutes. Manual delivery was attempted but was unsuccessful due to abnormal adherence.

6 A 28-year-old G5 P. 4 woman has an uneventful pregnancy. Her fetal morphology scan at 20 weeks was normal and the placenta noted as fundal in position. She had a spontaneous vaginal delivery at 37 weeks and the placenta was delivered with a gush of blood and lengthening of the cord. However, the bleeding did not stop and she lost over 800 mL of blood. A red bulging mass is noted at the introitus.

a Phenytoin

b Warfarin

c Fluoextine

d Labetolol

e Diazepam

f Lamotrigine

g Heparin

h Imipramine

i Ramipril

j Aspirin

Some medications can cause profound effects on the neonate. Match the following scenarios with the possible answers. Answers may be used once, more than once or not at all.

7 A medication which can cause neonatal renal failure, hypotension, oligohydramnios and intra-uterine death.

8 A medication that can cause cleft lip and palate, and septal heart defects.

9 A medication that causes 'floppy baby syndrome'.

10 A medication that causes saddle nose, frontal bossing, short stature and mental retardation.

11 A medication causing muscle spasms, irritability and tachycardia.

12 A medication that can cause progressive encephalitis and a fatty liver.

a   Psoriasis

b   *Pediculosis pubis*

c   Behçet's syndrome

d   Eczema

e   Hypertrophic dystrophy

f   Bullous pemphigoid

g   Primary atrophy

h   Lichen planus

i   Vulval carcinoma

j   Hairy leukoplakia

k   Diabetes mellitus

l   Hypothyroidism

m   Lymphoma

n   *Sarcoptes scabei*

o   Lichen sclerosus et atrophicus

For each of the following scenarios concerning vulval conditions, choose the diagnosis from the list of options above. Each option may be used once, more than once or not at all.

13   An 18-year-old woman presents with pruritis in the vulval region. There is no vaginal discharge. She recently had unprotected sexual intercourse.

14   A 60-year-old woman presents with vulval pruritis, which is disturbing her sleep. On examination you note ivory coloured thickened skin that extends onto the thighs and perineum.

15   A 78-year-old woman presents with intense vulval pruritus. On examination you note irregular white patches on the inner aspects of the labia majora. Only the genitalia are involved.

16   A 50-year-old woman presents with dyspareunia and vulval soreness. On examination the vulval skin is red and shiny as are the vaginal walls. No skin thickening is seen. The introitus is contracted.

17   A 35-year-old obese woman suffers from recurrent vulval pruritis and a thick white discharge.

   a Stillbirth

   b Late fetal loss

   c Early neonatal death

   d Late neonatal death

   e Post-neonatal death

Use one of the above options to define each of the following scenarios relating to mortality. Each option may be used once, more than once or not at all.

18 A fetus is known to have died in utero at 22 weeks, but is delivered at 25 weeks.

19 An infant dies 30 days after birth.

20 An infant dies at the age of six months.

21 A baby dies at the age of 10 days.

a Prolactinoma

b Hypothyroidism

c Exercise induced

d Sheehan's syndrome

e Asherman's syndrome

f PCOS

g Premature ovarian failure

h Pregnancy

i Climacteric

Match the following scenarios with the causes for amenorrhoea and oligomenorrhea. Each option may be used once, more than once or not at all

22 A 38-year-old woman with amenorrhoea complains of headaches, peripheral visual loss and galactorrhca.

23 A 25-year-old woman presents with recent onset oligomenorrhea and galactorrhea. She denies any other symptoms. Her pregnancy test is negative. She has a past history of radioisotope treatment for Grave's disease.

24 A 27-year-old woman had a vaginal delivery 12 months ago complicated by severe postpartum haemorrhage. She was unable to breastfeed and has not had a period since her pregnancy. A pregnancy test is negative.

25 A 50-year-old woman presents with longer intervals between her periods for the past eight months, night sweats, difficulty sleeping and vaginal dryness.

26 A 32-year-old woman complains of amenorrhoea since she had a dilatation and curettage for an incomplete miscarriage. She denies any other symptoms and an examination carried out was normal.

a   Arrange fetal blood sampling

b   Reassurance

c   Expedite delivery

d   Stop syntocinon

e   Give 500 mL crystalloid

f   Attach fetal scalp electrode

g   Lay on left lateral side

h   Discontinue continuous fetal monitoring

i   Give tocolysis

j   Repeat fetal blood sampling within 30 minutes or consider delivery if rapid fall in pH since last sample

k   Continue monitoring and repeat fetal blood sampling within one hour or sooner if fetal heart rate abnormalities persist

For each of the following scenarios relating to intrapartum fetal monitoring, choose one management option from the list above. Each option may be used once, more than once or not at all.

27 A multiparous woman with previous Caesarean section is in the first stage of labour. Her labour has not progressed well. Fetal CTG shows reduced variability for 90 minutes with normal baseline and variable decelerations. A fetal blood sample pH value is 7.27.

28 A primiparous woman is having continuous fetal monitoring as labour is not progressing well and a syntocinon infusion has been commenced. CTG shows much 'loss of contact' although the uterine contractions are well established.

29 A primiparous woman is in labour and despite syntocinon has not progressed well. The CTG shows reduced variability over 90 minutes, baseline has risen to 170 bpm and there is a prolonged deceleration lasting three minutes.

30 A multiparous woman is in the first stage of labour, progressing well. She has no previous adverse obstetric history. CTG shows normal features.

SINGLE BEST ANSWER: FOR EACH QUESTION CHOOSE ONE ANSWER ONLY

1 According to the March 2008 NICE guidelines for diabetes in pregnancy, what is the recommended level for fasting blood glucose for women who are pregnant?

   a 3.5–5.9 mmol/L

   b 4–6.5 mmol/L

   c 8–6.8 mmol/L

   d 4.5–7.0 mmol/L

   e 4.5–.9 mmol/L

2 According to the October 2006 NICE guidelines for urinary incontinence, for what minimum time period should pelvic floor muscle training be undertaken for stress or mixed urinary incontinence?

   a Two weeks

   b Four weeks

   c Two months

   d Three months

   e Six months

3 The correct advice for wearing a three point car seatbelt whilst pregnant is:

   a Use a lap belt only

   b The belt should be under the bump

   c The belt should be over the bump

   d The belt should be above and below the bump

   e Not to wear a seatbelt

4 Which ONE of the following conditions does NOT have malignant potential?

   a Paget's disease

   b Moniliasis

   c Melanoma in situ

   d Lichen sclerosus

   e Leukoplakia

5 Risk factors for placental abruption include all of the following EXCEPT:

   a Pre-eclampsia

   b Smoking

   c Oligohydramnios

   d Multiparity

   e Road traffic accident

6 After how much time are the long-acting reversible contraceptives more cost effective than the combined oral pill?

   a Three months

   b Six months

   c One year

   d Two years

   e They are not more cost effective

7 A baby is born to a mother who has had an emergency Caesarean section due to placental abruption at 35 weeks. He is pale, taking irregular breaths and is showing slight flexion of his limbs. His heart rate is 95 bpm and he grimaces on reflex. What is his Apgar score?

   a 1

   b 2

   c 3

   d 4

   e 5

8 How much folic acid per day is recommended for a pregnant lady with coeliac disease?

   a 0.4 mg

   b 0.5 mg

   c 1 mg

   d 3 mg

   e 5 mg

9 If simple measures have failed, the recommended treatment for seborrhoeic dermatits is:

a Olive oil applied to baby's scalp

b Baby shampoo

c Antifungal cream

d Steroid cream

e Steroid scalp treatment

10 Concerning parity and gravidity how would you express a pregnant lady who has three children: two boys aged 14 and 8 years, and a girl aged 12 years. She also had one stillbirth at 29 weeks and two miscarriages at 16 and 18 weeks, respectively, as well as one ectopic pregnancy at 8 weeks:

a G8 P. 4+3

b G8 P. 3+3

c G7 P. 4+3

d G8 P. 3+4

e G7 P. 4+4

11 The effects of smoking while pregnant include all of the following EXCEPT:

a Pre-term labour

b Placenta praevia

c Stillbirth and miscarriages

d Placental abruption

e Pre-eclampsia

12 Indications for amniocentesis include all of the following EXCEPT:

a Advanced maternal age

b A previous child with chromosomal abnormalities

c Mothers exposed to certain drugs or infections that may cause fetal malformations

d Mothers carrying X-linked disorder to determine fetal sex

e Screening for neural tube defect

13 Which ONE feature is NOT included in the diagnostic criteria for fetal alcohol syndrome?

   a Maternal drinking

   b Characteristic facial anomalies

   c Chromosomal defect

   d Central nervous system neurodevelopmental anomalies

   e Growth restriction

14 An 18-year-old patient presents to your GP practice with shoulder tip pain. On closer questioning she has had a history of amenorrhoea for seven weeks. On examination she is tender in her RIF, but denies any vaginal bleed. Her urine pregnancy test comes back positive. What is your further management?

   a Confirm with blood ßhCG and repeat in 48 hours to see if doubles

   b Order an ultrasound scan

   c Admit to the emergency department

   d Abdominal ultrasound to exclude gall stones

   e Provide ante-natal advise and recommend folic acid

15 Which ONE of the following factors reduces the likelihood of Caesarean section?

   a Planned delivery in a midwifery-led unit for healthy women with uncomplicated pregnancy

   b Electronic fetal monitoring

   c Home delivery for healthy women with uncomplicated pregnancy

   d Non supine position during the second stage

   e Walking in labour

16 Which ONE of the following statements is NOT true regarding urethral caruncles?

   a They are always solitary.

   b They usually cause symptoms.

   c They usually occur in postmenopausal women.

   d They arise from the anterior wall of the urethra.

   e They are not neoplastic.

17 Pre-eclampsia is pregnancy-induced hypertension in association with how much proteinuria?

a   0.1 g in 24 hours

b   0.3 g in 24 hours

c   0.5 g in 24 hours

d   3 g in 24 hours

e   5 g in 24 hours

18 After how many UTIs in a year may a woman be referred for further investigation?

a   One

b   Two

c   Three

d   Four

e   Five

Examination C
PAPER 1 ANSWERS

EXTENDED MATCHING QUESTIONS

1 f

2 b

3 c

Red degeneration is treated conservatively with bed rest, analgesia and fluids. The acute symptoms subside over one to two weeks and the pregnancy usually proceeds normally.

Ovarian torsion in pregnancy is treated by laparotomy and untwisting the ovary, if still viable, or by oophorectomy.

Risk factors for placental abruption include a past history, high blood pressure, trauma, multiple pregnancies, high parity, polyhydramnios, short umbilical cord and smoking/alcohol/cocaine use.

4 c

5 e

6 d

Uterine atony is the most common cause of PPH and unlike retained products of conception there is no crampy pain associated with the bleed. It complicates approximately 1 in 20 births. Causes include over-distension (including polyhydramnios, macrosomia and twins), drugs and uterine fatigue from prolonged labour. First-line therapy should be uterine massage.

The risk factors for placenta accreta increase from 5% in a uterus not exposed to procedures to 25% in a uterus that has undergone a Caesarean section. Other risk factors include placenta praevia, D+C and grandmultiparity.

Risk factors include higher parity, a fundal placenta, placenta accreta and other abnormally adherent placentas, placenta praevia and connective tissue diseases (e.g. Marfan's syndrome).

7 i

8 a

9 e

10 b

11 h

12 j

British National Formulary. London: BMJ Publishing Group; 2008.

13 b

14 o

15 e

16 g

17 k

Pediculosis pubis, or pubic lice are transmitted by close contact and cause pubic itching. Treatment involves contact tracing, malathion and a full STD screen.

In lichen sclerosus, intensely itchy areas of slightly thickened (hyperkeratotic) skin are found on the genitalia and may extend into the thighs and perineum. It may respond to steroid creams. Hypertrophic dystrophy occurs in previously atrophic areas, confined to the labia, introitus and clitoris most commonly; these are also the more common sites of cancer. Treat with topical steroids or bland ointments. These disorders have malignant potential so sufferers require follow-up.

Atrophy is most common around the climacteric due to reducing levels of oestrogen in the body. Treat with topical oestrogens or topical steroids. Follow-up is essential as hypertrophic changes, which have malignant potential, may occur/systemic oestrogen side effects.

Don't forget systemic disease may present with dermatological symptoms. Diabetes should be excluded in anyone with recurrent thrush.

18 b

19 e

20 e

21 d

Late fetal loss: An in utero death between 22+0 and 23+6 weeks' gestation. According to the RCOG good practice guideline 'Registration
of stillbirths and certification of pregnancy loss before 24 weeks of
gestation', if a fetus dies in utero before 24 weeks, but is expelled after
24 weeks, it is not registered as a stillbirth, but classed as a fetal loss,
or miscarriage.

Royal College of Obstetricians and Gynaecologists. *Registration of
Stillbirths and Certification of Pregnancy Loss Before 24 Weeks of Gestation:
RCOG good practice no. 4.* London: Royal College of Obstetricians and
Gynaecologists; 2005.

Stillbirth: Any 'child' expelled or issued forth by its mother after
the 24th week of pregnancy that did not breathe or show any other
signs of life.

Early neonatal death: Death of a live born baby occurring less
than seven completed days from the time of birth.

Late neonatal death: Death of a live born baby occurring after the
7th day and before 28 completed days from the time of birth.

Post-neonatal death: Death from age 28 days to 1 year.

Infant death: All deaths from birth to age one year.

www.statistics.gov.uk

22 a

23 b

24 d

25 i

26 e

Treatment involves bromocriptine to reduce the size of the pituitary
adenoma if large followed by surgery.

The cause of hyperprolactinaemia in hypothyroid patients is
undetermined. One school of thought suggests TRH, which stimulates TSH, also stimulates prolactin secretion; the other school of
thought maybe that hypothyroid patients have a decreased ability to
excrete prolactin.

Severe PPH and inability to breast feed suggest anterior pituitary
failure.

27 k

28 f

29 c

30 h

The table below gives the current NICE guidance on appropriate responses to fetal scalp pH results.

Fetal blood sample (FBS) result/pH	Subsequent action
≥7.25	Repeat FBS in one hour if fetal heart rate abnormalities persist
7.21–7.24	Repeat FBS within 30 minutes or consider delivery if rapid fall in pH since last sample
<7.20	Delivery indicated

All fetal scalp blood pH estimations should be interpreted taking into account the previous pH measurement, the rate of progress in labour and the clinical features of the mother and baby. Where continuous monitoring is indicated and the CTG is of poor quality, a fetal scalp electrode should be attached with maternal consent. A prolonged deceleration is an indicator of acute fetal compromise. Fetal blood sampling is not indicated, delivery is. Continuous monitoring of fetal heart rate in normal labour is not advised.

National Institute for Health and Clinical Excellence. *Intrapartum Care: management and delivery of care to women in labour: NICE guideline 55*. London: NIHCE; 2007. www.nice.org.uk/guidance/CG055

SINGLE BEST ANSWER

1 a

They also advise that the one-hour post-prandial blood glucose should be below 7.8 mmol/L.

2 d

3 d

National Institute for Health and Clinical Excellence. *Antenatal Care: routine care for the healthy pregnant woman: NICE guideline 62*. London: NIHCE; 2008. www.nice.org.uk/guidance/CG062

4 b

Moniliasis is thrush. Leukoplakia is also called hypertrophic dystrophy. Vulval intraepithelial neoplasia also has malignant potential.

5 c

Other risk factors include: polyhydramnios, previous abruption, trauma including iatrogenic (e.g. external cephalic version) and thrombophilia.

6 c

According to the NICE guideline for long-acting reversible contraception October 2005 they are cost effective after one year.

National Institute for Health and Clinical Excellence. *Long-Acting Reversible Contraception: the effective and appropriate use of long-acting reversible contraception: NICE guideline 30.* London: NIHCE; 2005. www.nice.org.uk/guidance/CG030

7 d

8 e

The Department of Health recommends 0.4 mg daily for normal pregnancy, and 5 mg for ladies on epileptic medication, mothers who have had a previous pregnancy complicated by a neural tube defect or a partner or first degree relative with a spinal cord defect, coeliac disease (due to malabsorption), sickle cell disease or thalassemia. The supplement should be taken before conception till 13 weeks gestation.

9 c

Seborrhoeic dermatitis is a benign and self-limiting common neonatal problem. Known to be fungal in nature, it usually responds to simple measures like softening the scales with oil and shampooing off but may need topical antifungal (e.g. ketoconazole 2% cream or shampoo for a few weeks to clear).

www.cks.library.nhs.uk/seborrhoeic_dermatitis

10 a

Gravidity refers to the number of pregnancies to any stage including the present one. Parity is written as X+Y: X is the number of pregnancies resulting in live or stillbirths and Y the number of losses before 24 weeks (e.g. termination, spontaneous abortions, ectopics or moles). Successful twin pregnancies are expressed as G1 P. 2; that is, one pregnancy with twins (2X). If a patient has two miscarriages under 24 weeks gestation it is expressed as G2 P. 0+2.

11 e

Initially, the mother should be encouraged to stop smoking with counselling and behavioural therapies. However, if these fail, the lowest dose and duration of nicotine replacement therapy (so as to reduce nicotine exposure to the fetus) can be used. Champix® and Zyban® are contraindicated.

A case control study of primigravidae who smoke as compared to non-smokers suggests a decreasing relative risk of pre-eclampsia and gestational hypertension with increasing daily smoking habits.

Marcoux S, Brisson J, Fabia J. The effect of cigarette smoking on the risk of pre-eclampsia and gestational hypertension. *Am J Epidemiol.* 1989; **130**(5): 950–7.

12 e

Amniocentesis is not used as a screening tool, but is used after positive ante-natal tests, for example, ultrasound or raised alpha feta protein, for confirmation. The fluid obtained during amniocentesis contains both fetal and maternal cells and may be used in the management of Rhesus disease or estimating maturity. The cells undergo chromosomal, genetic, biochemical and biological analysis; for example, bilirubin for assessment and detection of isoimmune haemolysis, alpha feta protein and acetylcholinesterase levels for neural tube defects, lecithin to sphingomyelin ratio to assess lung maturity and DNA tests on fetal cells (e.g. to detect Fragile X, sickle cell disease or cystic fibrosis).

13 c

This is a common disorder and takes the form of a spectrum. Most ante-natal care happens in the community and we should ask women throughout their pregnancy about their drinking habits. Diagnostic criteria for fetal alcohol syndrome:

1 Confirmed maternal alcohol exposure

2 Characteristic facial anomalies that include short palpebral fissures, abnormalities in the premaxillary zone (e.g. flat upper lip, flattened philtrum and flat midface)

3 Evidence of growth restriction in at least one of the following:
   - low birth weight for gestational age
   - decelerating weight over time not due to nutrition
   - disproportionally low weight to height

4 Evidence of central nervous system neurodevelopmental abnormalities, at least one of the following:

- decreased cranial size at birth
- structural brain abnormalities (e.g. microcephaly, partial or complete agenesis of the corpus callosum, cerebellar hypoplasia)
- neurological hard or soft signs (as age appropriate) such as impaired fine motor skills, neurosensory hearing loss, poor tandem gait, poor eye–hand coordination

Stratton K, Howe C, Battaglia F, editors. *Fetal Alcohol Syndrome: diagnosis, epidemiology, prevention, and treatment.* Washington, DC: National Academies Press; 1996.

14 c

The patient has an ectopic pregnancy unless proved otherwise. Not all patients present with the classical prune juice discharge prior to pain.

15 c

Delivery in a midwifery-led unit does not reduce the likelihood of Caesarean section, but home delivery does.

National Institute for Health and Clinical Excellence. *Caesarean Section: NICE guideline 13.* London: NIHCE; 2004. www.nice.org.uk/guidance/CG013

16 d

A urethral caruncle arises from the posterior wall of the urethra and is thought to be due to chronic infection of the paraurethral glands in the floor. They can be asymptomatic but commonly cause pain, bleeding or dysuria. Treatment is by excision/diathermy.

www.gpnotebook.co.uk

17 b

18 c

Recurrent UTI is defined as three or more in a year. These women should be investigated for any underlying cause, such as a renal tract abnormality. However, if there is an obvious trigger such as coitus, it may be felt that further investigations are not warranted for simple UTIs. Recurrent infection should be documented with a culture.

Car J, Sheikh A. Recurrent urinary tract infection in women: ten-minute consultation. *BMJ.* 2003; **327:** 1204.

Examination C
PAPER 2

MULTIPLE CHOICE QUESTIONS

1 Fetal nuchal translucency:
   a Is performed between 11 weeks and 13 weeks plus six days
   b Decreased thickness may reflect heart failure
   c Is strongly associated with chromosomal abnormalities
   d Is a diagnostic test
   e Combined with noting the presence or absence of fetal nasal bone increases sensitivity of Down's syndrome detection

2 The following women should be offered elective Caesarean section:
   a Women with Hepatitis B infection
   b HIV-positive women
   c Pregnant women with a recurrence of genital HSV infection at birth
   d Women with Hepatitis C infection
   e Women co-infected with Hepatitis C and HIV

3 Non-contraceptive effects of the oral contraceptives.
   a The combined oral pill reduces the incidence of tubal infertility.
   b The combined oral pill increases the risk of ectopic pregnancy.
   c The POP increases the risk of ectopic pregnancy.
   d The combined oral pill increases the risk of ovarian cancer.
   e The combined oral pill reduces the risk of benign breast disease.

4 Regarding perinatal mortality.

   a The perinatal mortality rate is defined as the number of stillbirths and early neonatal deaths per 1000 live births.

   b The neonatal mortality rate is defined as the number of neonatal deaths per 1000 live births.

   c The neonatal mortality rate has reached a plateau.

   d Stillbirth, perinatal mortality and neonatal deaths are all more common in mothers aged under 20 years or over 40 years.

   e The stillbirth rate in the UK is around 5 per 1000 total births.

5 Cri-du-chat syndrome is associated with the following:

   a Deletion of the short arm of chromosome 6

   b Microcephaly

   c Closely-spaced eyes

   d Cardiovascular problems

   e 'Moon' face

6 Chickenpox in pregnancy.

   a It is infectious 72 hours prior to the rash appearing and until the last spot has crusted over.

   b If a pregnant woman comes into contact with chickenpox a blood test should be carried out to confirm varicella zoster immunity.

   c Varicella zoster immunoglobulin (VZIG) is effective up to seven days post exposure.

   d A second dose of VZIG is not effective if a second exposure occurs.

   e Herpes zoster (shingles) cannot be transmitted to a pregnant woman from close contact.

7 Causes for an abnormal sperm analysis include:

   a Tight under garments

   b Smoking

   c Alcohol

   d Recreational drugs

   e Cold weather

8 Down's syndrome is associated with the following:

   a Muscle hypertonia

   b Protruding tongue

   c Single palmar crease

   d Central silver iris spots (Brushfield's spots)

   e Flat facial profile

9 Concerning treatment for fibroids.

   a Laparoscopic myomectomy is the best surgical option for women with fibroids who want to preserve their fertility.

   a Uterine artery embolisation (UAE) is a safe option for women who want to preserve their fertility.

   b UAE results in better improvement in pelvic pain than hysterectomy.

   c There is a higher risk of bleeding with open hysterectomy than with laparoscopic techniques.

   d GnRH agonists can produce a reduction in size of fibroids up to 50%.

10 Antihypertensive medications recommended for use in pregnancy are:

   a Atenolol

   b Labetolol

   c Hydralazine

   d Ramipril

   e Bendrofluazide

11 Complications of oligohydramnios:

   a Pulmonary hypoplasia

   b Breech presentation

   c Amniotic band syndrome

   d Talipes eqinovarus

   e Macrosomia

12 HSV type 2 infection.

   a It usually presents with a solitary painful ulcer.

   b Treatment is useless if started after 48 hours of onset of symptoms.

   c The primary attack tends to be the shortest and least painful.

   d Neonatal HSV encephalitis may occur.

   e Asymptomatic viral shedding reduces over time.

13 Concerning fetal hydrops.

   a All pregnancies are non-viable leading to stillbirth.

   b Fifth disease (parvovirus B19) is a cause.

   c It is a severe manifestation of haemolytic disease.

   d Ascites, pleural and pericardial effusion and skin oedema may be present.

   e In all cases treatment includes intra uterine fetal transfusion with packed red cells.

14 Ovarian cancer can present with the following:

   a Urinary frequency

   b Pelvic mass

   c Amenorrhoea

   d Constipation

   e Abdominal bloating

15 Concerning placental abruption.

   a Unless the mother is in shock it can be managed in the community.

   b It is a risk factor for post-partum haemorrhage.

   c It always presents with blood loss and pain.

   d It requires anti-D if Rhesus-positive mother and Rhesus-negative father.

   e If concealed it is usually associated with a worse outcome than if revealed.

16 The risk of developing cervical cancer:
   a Is increased by current use of combined oral contraceptives (COCs) for more than 3 years
   b Is diminished to that of never users if the COC is stopped for 10 years
   c Is similar for COCs and progesterone-only injectable contraceptives
   d The number of extra cases of cervical cancer in COC users increases with age
   e Is decreased by using the progesterone releasing intrauterine system (IUS)

17 The following are associated with preterm delivery:
   a Polyhydramnios
   b Smoking
   c Pre-eclampsia
   d Afro-Caribbean race
   e Bacterial vaginosis

18 Syndromes associated with a decreased intelligence are:
   a Kleinfelter's syndrome
   b Turner's syndrome
   c Down's syndrome
   d Lesch-Nyhan syndrome
   e Noonan's syndrome

19 Illicit abuse of opiate drugs in pregnancy is associated with the following:
   a Antepartum haemorrhage
   b IUGR
   c Premature delivery
   d Neonatal withdrawal syndrome
   e Congenital anomalies

20 Management of PCOS.

    a Lifestyle modifications play no factor in aiding fertility.

    b With respect to infertility treatment, clomifene increases the risk of multiple pregnancies.

    c The combined oral contraceptive pill can be used.

    d Metformin is seen as the most important treatment of insulin resistance.

    e Spironolactone has anti-androgenic properties and decreases hirsutism.

21 Regarding breech presentation and ECV.

    a ECV has success rates of between 50–80%.

    b ECV in multiparous women is more successful.

    c Presenting part below the pelvic brim increases chances of success.

    d If the fetal heart rate falls below 100 bpm the procedure should be abandoned.

    e The Term Breech Trial found that planned vaginal delivery was no more hazardous than elective Caesarean section.

22 Endometriosis is more common in women who are:

    a Nulliparous

    b Caucasian

    c Afro-Caribbean

    d Of high social class

    e Overweight

23 Regarding perineal trauma.

    a A woman's physical and psychological health may be affected long term.

    b Urinary problems are more common than faecal incontinence long term.

    c Around 20% of women experience superficial dyspareunia up to three months post-delivery.

    d 70% of women experience pain up to 10 days post delivery.

    e Up to 10% of women can experience long-term pain (months).

24 The hypothalamic pituitary ovarian axis.

   a Pulsed release of FSH and LH occur from the posterior pituitary.

   b Both the Graafian follicle and the corpus luteum produce oestrogen and progesterone.

   c Production of steroids from the corpus luteum can be maintained by human chorionic gonadotropin from the implanting pregnancy until the 9th to 10th week when the placenta takes over steroid production.

   d Frequency of pulsed GnRH is decreased by increasing levels of oestrogen, towards the end of the follicular phase.

   e The release of FSH from the pituitary is directly reduced by inhibin.

25 The following are non-reassuring features of a fetal CTG:

   a Increase in baseline to 165 bpm

   b Variability <5 bpm for 60 minutes

   c Sinusoidal baseline for 15 minutes

   d Single prolonged deceleration lasting two minutes

   e Presence of accelerations

26 First trimester (11–13 weeks plus 6 days gestation) ante-natal screening tests for Down's syndrome include:

   a Nuchal translucency (NT) scan

   b The combined test: NT, maternal serum ßhCG and pregnancy-associated plasma protein-A (PAPP-A)

   c The triple test: maternal serum alpha fetal protein (αFP), ßhCG and unconjugated oestriol (uE3)

   d The quadruple test: maternal serum αFP, ßhCG, inhibin A and uE3

   e The double test: maternal serum αFP and ßhCG

27 Fetal blood sampling during labour:
    a Is always indicated for a pathological fetal cardiotocograph
    b Is undertaken with the mother lying on her back
    c Can be taken if there is a breech presentation
    d Is contraindicated in prematurity (<34 weeks)
    e Should be acted upon solely on the basis of the pH result

28 Human Papilloma Virus (HPV).
    a Subtypes 16 and 18 are associated with cancerous change.
    b Gardasil® vaccine is a bivalent vaccine.
    c Cervarix® is the chosen vaccine for national immunisation in the UK.
    d Vaccines utilise HPV virus-like particles to induce an antibody response and seroconvert the individual.
    e Subtypes 6 and 11 cause genital warts.

29 Higher rates of failure in operative (instrumental, assisted) vaginal delivery occur when:
    a Fetal head is above ischial spines
    b Fetal presentation is occipito-anterior
    c Maternal BMI is >30
    d The midwife is performing the procedure
    e Estimated fetal weight is >4 kg

30 Causes of secondary amenorrhoea include:
    a PCOS
    b Sheehan's syndrome
    c Bulimia
    d Lactation
    e Congenital adrenal hyperplasia

31 Care of a newborn.

  a The baby is best placed skin to skin with the mother as soon as possible post-delivery.

  b The baby loses a lot of heat through conduction when the skin is dry.

  c Hypothermia may worsen hypoxia and hypoglycaemia.

  d If the baby has irregular breaths at birth immediate resuscitation with a mask is necessary.

  e If meconium is seen at the vocal cords then intubation is usually necessary.

32 Choriocarcinoma.

  a 50% follow previous molar pregnancies.

  b 25% follow previous ectopic or normal pregnancies.

  c Serum ßhCG is used to monitor treatment.

  d The success rate of treatment is 90% if no metastasis is present.

  e Radiotherapy may be used for metastases to lung or brain.

33 Regarding Caesarean section.

  a The risk of fetal lacerations is around 0.5%.

  b The risk of postoperative infection is 3%.

  c The risk of urinary tract injury is around 1%.

  d Wound dressing may be removed after 24 hours.

  e The risk of post-natal depression is significantly higher than after vaginal delivery.

34 Complications of surgical TOP are:

  a Uterine perforation

  b Asherman's syndrome

  c Breast cancer

  d Pelvic inflammatory disease

  e Ectopic pregnancy

35 Breast feeding.

  a Breast feeding can reduce the risk of necrotising enterocolitis (NEC) in pre-term babies.

  b Hormones, enzymes and immunoglobulins are all present in breast milk.

  c If a baby has phenylketonuria it is best to restrict the intake of breast milk.

  d If the mother has tuberculosis it is best not to breast feed.

  e HIV-positive mothers should be encouraged not to breastfeed to reduce transmission rates.

36 Beneficial treatment for symptoms of pre-menstrual syndrome:

  a Agnus castus

  b St John's Wort

  c Vitamin B6

  d Microgynon®

  e Yasmin®

37 Possible causes of prolonged neonatal jaundice (over 14 days):

  a Hypothyroidism

  b Infection

  c Cystic fibrosis

  d Biliary atresia

  e 'Breast milk' jaundice

38 Ectopic pregnancy.

  a Abdominal pain always precedes bleeding, which is classically 'prune juice'.

  b If female is Rhesus-negative and male Rhesus-positive they will require Anti-D injection.

  c The treatment of choice is surgical with laparotomy and salpingectomy.

  d Methotrexate treatment is always successful due to its function of inhibiting DNA synthesis.

  e Cornual ectopic pregnancies can only be diagnosed in approximately 70 % of cases by ultrasound.

39 With respect to uterine inversion.

  a It occurs in approximately 1 in 5000 deliveries.

  b The Brandt-Andrews method of delivery has been shown to increase the risk of uterine inversion.

  c Fundal implantation of the placenta is a risk factor.

  d It may present with shock out of proportion to blood loss.

  e Syntometrine is used prior to replacement.

40 *Chlamydia trachomatis*:

  a Can be isolated from urine

  b Has been the subject of national screening since 2000

  c Is the most common curable sexually transmitted infection in the UK

  d Infection may resolve spontaneously

  e 70% of women are asymptomatic

Examination C
PAPER 2 ANSWERS

MULTIPLE CHOICE

1 T, F, T, F, T

Nuchal translucency is assessed as the maximum thickness of the nuchal pad at the nape of the fetal neck. It varies with crown-rump length and gestational age. Three in four babies with Down's syndrome do not have a visible nasal bone at the time of first trimester screening. Increased nuchal translucency is also seen in anomalies of heart and greater arteries as well as heart failure.

2 F, T, F, F, T

Babies of women with Hepatitis B infection are given immunoglobulin and are vaccinated. There is insufficient evidence to say Caesarean section delivery reduces the risk of vertical transmission. HIV and co-infection of HIV with Hepatitis C is an indication for Caesarean section delivery. Primary genital HSV infection in the third trimester is an indication, but there is uncertainty regarding the effect of Caesarean section on neonatal HSV in women with a recurrence of genital HSV infection.

National Institute for Health and Clinical Excellence. *Caesarean Section: NICE guideline 13*. London: NIHCE; 2004. www.nice.org.uk/guidance/CG013

Vertical transmission of Hepatitis C is dependent on the level of viraemia in the mother, not the mode of delivery.

National Institutes of Health. *Management of hepatitis C. National Institutes of Health Consensus Conference Statement*. 10–12 June 2002. Bethesda, MA. http://consensus.nih.gov

3 T, F, T, F, T

The COCP protects against pelvic inflammatory disease and thus reduces the risk of tubal infertility and ectopic pregnancy. Due to the fact that the progesterone-only pill affects tubal migration of the egg and sperm, this can lead to an ectopic pregnancy, even though overall there is less risk of falling pregnant. The COCP reduces the risk of ovarian, endometrial cancer and benign breast disease.

4 F, T, F, T, F
The perinatal mortality rate is defined as the number of stillbirths and early neonatal deaths per 1000 live births and stillbirths. The neonatal mortality rate is defined as the number of neonatal deaths per 1000 live births. The neonatal mortality rate is declining; the stillbirth rate has reached a plateau. Maternal age, obesity and social deprivation are all demographic factors affecting perinatal mortality, stillbirth and neonatal mortality. The stillbirth rate is 5.3 per 1000 total births; the neonatal mortality rate is 3.4 per 1000 live births; and the perinatal mortality rate is 7.9 per 1000 total births.

Confidential Enquiry into Maternal and Child Health (CEMACH). *Perinatal Mortality 2006*. London: Confidential Enquiry into Maternal and Child Health; 2008.

5 F, T, F, T, T
Cri-du-chat syndrome is due to the deletion of the short arm of chromosome 5. Wide-spaced eyes and a high-pitched cry are characteristic.

6 F, T, F, F, F
Chickenpox is infectious 48 hours prior to the rash appearing. VZIG should be given to non-immune women who have a significant contact with chickenpox. It is effective up to 10 days post-contact. Blood tests usually take 24–48 hours to process and may be carried out on serum saved from routine ante-natal bloods. If necessary, a second VZIG dose can be given if a second exposure occurs and more than three months has elapsed from the previous dosage. The risk of contracting herpes zoster from a non-exposed rash (e.g. on the back) is very low; however, it is more risky if the rash is exposed. VZIG is given to prevent the development of chickenpox after exposure; it has no effect after the rash appears. Aciclovir is to be used if the woman presents up to 48 hours after the rash occurs. It is known to improve the length of fever and the rash, but has no statistical evidence to show a significant effect on the complication rate. Any woman who is at risk of pneumonitis (e.g. a smoker, an immunocompromised patient or those who have chronic obstructive lung disease), should be considered for a

referral to the hospital. Fetal varicella syndrome (FVS) does not occur after 28 weeks gestation.

Royal College of Obstetricians and Gynaecologists. *Chickenpox in Pregnancy: green-top 13*. London: Royal College of Obstetricians and Gynaecologists; 2007. www.rcog.org.uk

7 T, T, T, T, F

Heat and poor lifestyle issues will affect the quality of sperm. It is usually beneficial if the external genitalia are kept at a cooler temperature. If an abnormal test is received it is better to repeat the test at an interval of four to six weeks. Three tests should be carried out prior to deciding that there is sufficient evidence to refer for specialist input.

8 F, T, T, F, T

Muscle hypotonia is characteristic. A round head with a flat facial profile, dysplastic ears, blunt inner eye angles, broad hands with a single palmar crease and an incurving 5th digit are other features of Down's syndrome. Brushfield's spots are on the periphery of the iris.

9 T, F, F, F, T

www.patient.co.uk

National Institute for Health and Clinical Excellence. *Uterine Artery Embolisation for the Treatment of Fibroids: NICE Interventional Procedure Guidance 94*. London: NIHCE; 2004.
www.nice.org.uk/Guidance/IPG094

10 F, T, T, F, F

Atenolol, ACE inhibitors (e.g. such as ramipril) and diuretics (e.g. bendrofluazide), should be avoided in pregnancy.

Royal College of Obstetricians and Gynaecologists. *Management of Severe Eclampsia/Pre-Eclampsia: green-top 10A*. London: Royal College of Obstetricians and Gynaecologists; 2006. www.rcog.org.uk

11 T, T, T, T, F

Fetal mortality has been reported as high as 80–90% when oligohydramnios is diagnosed in the second trimester. This is generally due to major congenital malformation and pulmonary hypoplasia.

12 F, F, F, T, T

HSV type 2 affects the genitals most commonly however may cause oral sores as well. Usual presentation is with crops of vesicles or ulcers, may be bilateral. Primary attack is worst in severity and lasts the longest. Asymptomatic viral shedding is most likely in first 12 months.

Neonatal HSV features: blisters, jaundice, encephalitis, disseminated intravascular coagulation (DIC). Vertical transmission is most likely if first attack in third trimester. Can be acquired in utero as well. Treat with acyclovir 200 mg five times a day for five days, however treatment can be initiated within five days of symptom onset or later if new vesicles appearing. Aciclovir used in pregnancy but unlicensed, so get advice.

RCGP Sex, Drugs & HIV Task Group and BASHH. *Sexually Transmitted Infections in Primary Care*. London: RCGP; 2006.

13 F, T, T, T, F

Clinical features of fetal hydrops are due to fluid overload and include cardiac and respiratory failure, hepatosplenomegaly and generalised oedema. Investigations include tests to detect ante-natal antibodies against fetal red blood cells, screening for CMV, syphilis, rubella, toxoplasmosis and parvovirus B19 as well as genotyping (e.g. Turner's syndrome, and trisomies 13, 18 and 21 may be causes). Treatment depends on cause, with severely anaemic fetuses of isoimmunised pregnancies being treated with transfusion.

14 T, T, T, T, T

Ovarian cancer presentation is classically vague and non-specific. It is more common in postmenopausal women and can present with predominantly abdominal symptoms. NICE advises an urgent ultrasound if a woman presents with an unexplained abdominal or pelvic mass. If urgent ultrasound is not available locally, urgent referral is advised.

National Institute for Health and Clinical Excellence. *Referral for Suspected Cancer: NICE clinical guideline 27*. London: NIHCE; 2005. www.nice.org.uk/Guidance/CG27

15 F, T, F, F, T

There are two forms of placental abruption.

- Concealed – approximately 20% of cases where haemorrhage is confirmed within uterine cavity
- Revealed – 80%, which present with vaginal bleeding.

Symptoms are usually abdominal pain, a hard uterus and difficulty in palpating fetal parts. All women should be admitted for observation and fetal monitoring. Blood loss of less than 1000 mL leads to fetal hypoxia and distress, while over 1500 mL usually leads to maternal shock and fetal death. It may present with back ache, uterine hypercontractility and DIC. A concealed abruption may lead to maternal shock, renal failure and Sheehan's syndrome.

16 F, T, T, T, F

A 2007 Lancet paper examined data from >16 500 women with cervical cancer and found that current use of COCs for more than five years is accompanied by an increased risk of developing cervical cancer (relative risk 1.9). Stopping the pill for 10 years or more reduces the risk back down to that of never users. The risk is similar for COCs and progesterone-only injectable contraceptives (e.g. Depo-Provera®). However, no data are available on the risk with the IUS. The number of extra cases of cervical cancer in COC users increases with age and the number of years COCs are used.

International Collaboration of Epidemiological Studies of Cervical Cancer. Cervical cancer and hormonal contraceptives: collaborative reanalysis of individual data for 16 573 women with cervical cancer and 35 509 women without cervical cancer from 24 epidemiological studies. *Lancet.* 2007; **370**(9599): 1609–21.

www.cancerscreening.nhs.uk/cervical/drug-safety-update-april-2008.pdf

17 T, T, T, T, T

Other associations include excessive alcohol use, maternal age under 17 years or over 35 years, cervical incompetence, heroin withdrawal, multiple pregnancy and placental abruption.

www.patient.co.uk/showdoc/40024676/

18 T, F, T, T, T

Other examples include – Fragile X syndrome and Edward's syndrome.

19 T, T, T, T, F

There is no evidence that opiates cause congenital anomalies. Also cannabis, alcohol and opiates are all associated with premature delivery and IUGR. Cocaine abuse during pregnancy is associated with antepartum haemorrhage, preterm delivery, congenital abnormalities and intra-uterine growth restriction. Alcohol is associated with neurodevelopmental delay.

McCarthy A, Hunter B. *Obstetrics and Gynaecology: a core text with self-assessment.* Oxford: Churchill Livingstone; 1998.

20 F, T, T, F, T

Clomifene is an antioestrogen that blocks oestradiol binding to oestrogen receptors in the hypothalamus, thus preventing the negative feedback of FSH. The increase in FSH levels leads to an increase in ovarian follicles that are monitored via ultrasound to see a dominant follicle. Six per cent of people treated with clomifene have multiple pregnancies. Weight loss and exercise can stimulate ovulation and are the most important treatment of insulin resistance. COCP use increases sex hormone binding globulin and as such decreases free testosterone.

21 T, T, F, F, F

ECV should be offered to all uncomplicated breech pregnancies at 37 weeks according to NICE. It has a success rate of around 46–80%, which is improved if the presenting part is above the pelvic brim, and by multiparity, tocolysis and adequate liquor volume. ECV should only be carried out where facilities for continuous fetal monitoring, ultrasound and delivery by emergency Caesarean section are available. The procedure should be abandoned if the fetal heart rate drops below 90 bpm. The Term Breech Trial found that planned vaginal delivery is more hazardous than elective Caesarean section and for this reason women are offered delivery by the latter route. A planned Caesarean section reduced the relative risk of perinatal or neonatal mortality or serious neonatal morbidity by one-third. However, the methodology has been called into question.

Hannah ME, Hannah WJ, Hewson SA, *et al.*, Term Breech Trial Collaborative Group. Planned Caesarean section versus planned vaginal birth for breech presentation at term: a randomised multicentre trial. *Lancet.* 2000; **356**(9239): 1375–83.

National Institute for Health and Clinical Excellence. *Antenatal Care: routine care for the healthy pregnant woman: NICE clinical guideline 62.* London: NIHCE; 2008. www.nice.org.uk/guidance/CG055

22 T, T, F, T, F

Endometriosis is also common in women who start a family late in life, are underweight, are in the 30- to 40-year age group and are high achievers with Type A personalities.

23 T, T, T, F, T

Between 23% and 42% of women experience pain up to 10 days post delivery. Perineal trauma can be a significant cause of physical and psychological distress. It is important to empathise with patients and refer appropriately. Remember to ask about symptoms after the six-week post-natal check too as up to 1 in 10 women will still be experiencing pain 18 months post delivery. Around 3–10% report faecal incontinence at three months and around 24% report urinary problems.

Glazener CMA, Abdalla M, Stroud P, *et al*. Post-natal maternal morbidity: extent, causes, prevention and treatment. *Br J Obstet Gynaecol*. 1995; **102**(4): 282–7.

Sultan AH, Kamm MA, Hudson CN, *et al*. Anal sphincter disruption during vaginal delivery. *N Engl J Med*. 1993; **329**(26): 1905–11.

24 F, F, T, F, T

After puberty pulsed GnRH from the hypothalamus stimulates FSH and LH pulse release from the anterior pituitary. This is controlled by negative feedback of high levels of oestrogen, progesterone and inhibin on both the hypothalamus and pituitary. Frequency of pulsed GnRH is increased by oestrogen towards the end of follicular phase and decreased by progesterone and testosterone during the secretory phase until progesterone levels fall at the end of the cycle.

25 T, T, F, T, F

Feature of fetal heart rate trace	Baseline (bpm)	Variability (bpm)	Decelerations	Accelerations
Reassuring	110–60	≥5	None	Present
Non-reassuring	100–9 161–80	<for 40–90 minutes	Typical variable decelerations with over 50% of contractions, occurring for over 90 minutes	The absence of accelerations with otherwise normal trace is of uncertain significance
			Single prolonged deceleration for up to three minutes	
Abnormal	<100 >180 Sinusoidal pattern ≥10 minutes	<5 for 90 minutes	Either atypical variable decelerations with over 50% of contractions or late decelerations, both for over 30 minutes	
			Single prolonged deceleration for more than three minutes	

Normal: all four features are reassuring.

Suspicious: one non-reassuring feature, the rest reassuring.

Pathological: two or more features non reassuring or at least one abnormal feature.

National Institute for Health and Clinical Excellence. *Intrapartum Care: management and delivery of care to women in labour: NICE guideline 55*. London: NIHCE; 2007. www.nice.org.uk/guidance/CG055

26 T, T, F, F, F

NICE advises that all pregnant women should be offered screening for Down's Syndrome. At gestations between 11 weeks and 13 weeks plus 6 days, this should be in the form of the combined test (NT, ßhCG and PAPP-A). If booking late, or if fetal position/maternal BMI are obscuring the NT, then serum screening (i.e. triple/quadruple test) should be offered between 15 and 20 weeks gestation. The double test has been replaced by these. The triple test assesses the risk of having a baby with Down's syndrome by considering maternal age and maternal serum levels of αFP, ßhCG and uE3. A high ßhCG, low αFP and low uE3 suggest a Down's pregnancy. A high αFP suggests a neural tube defect. The quadruple test includes serum inhibin A as well, which improves screening sensitivity and specificity, but may not be available in all areas of the UK at present. Increasing maternal age is associated with an increased risk of having a baby with Down's syndrome: approximately 1 in 1500 at age 20, 1 in 270 at age 35 and ≥1 in 50 at age ≥45. Remember to counsel ALL women undergoing these tests regarding their pros/cons. Screening tests are NOT diagnostic – chorionic villus sampling (CVS) or amniocentesis is offered if indicated.

National Institute for Health and Clinical Excellence. *Antenatal Care: routine care for the healthy pregnant woman. NICE clinical guideline 62*. London: NIHCE; 2008. www.nice.org.uk/guidance/CG055

27 F, F, F, T, F

Fetal blood sampling (to ascertain scalp pH) is indicated for a pathological CTG in the absence of maternal and fetal contraindications, for example, fetal haemophilia, prematurity, maternal infection such as HIV, hepatitis and HSV, and unless there is evidence of acute fetal compromise. The mother should assume the left lateral position. FBS should not be undertaken for breech presentation. The result should not be acted upon solely; rather, other factors, such as overall condition of mother and baby, progress in labour and previous pH measurement, should be considered as well.

National Institute for Health and Clinical Excellence. *Intrapartum Care: management and delivery of care to women in labour: NICE guideline 55.* London: NIHCE; 2007. www.nice.org.uk/guidance/CG055

28 T, F, T, T, T

HPV subtypes 16 and 18 are associated with over 70% of cervical cancers. Subtypes 6 and 11 cause genital warts. Gardasil®, a quadrivalent vaccine, protects against serotypes 6, 11, 16 and 18. However, Cervarix®, a bivalent vaccine, protects against serotypes 16 and 18. An antibody response to the HPV subtype-specific virus-like particle seroconverts the individual and she is protected.

www.gpnotebook.co.uk

29 T, F, T, F, T

Occiput posterior (OP) position is associated with higher rates of failure in operative vaginal delivery, but there is no evidence to suggest that midwives are associated with higher failure rates.

Murphy DJ, Liebling RE, Verity L, *et al.* Early maternal and neonatal morbidity associated with operative delivery in second stage of labour: a cohort study. *Lancet.* 2001; **358**(9289): 1203–7.

Face presentation is contraindicated in ventouse extraction, not forceps. Fetal distress and lack of progress in the second stage as well as medical reasons for mother to avoid pushing (e.g. cardiac disease, myasthenia gravis) are indications for operative delivery.

Royal College of Obstetricians and Gynaecologists. *Operative Vaginal Delivery: green-top 26.* London: Royal College of Obstetricians and Gynaecologists; 2005. www.rcog.org.uk

30 T, T, T, T, F

Other causes of secondary amenorrhoea include: pregnancy, anovulation, menopause, hyperprolactinaemia, Asherman's syndrome, thyroid dysfunction, drug induced (e.g. Depo Provera®), haemochromatosis, exercise induced, stress and anorexia.

31 T, F, T, F, T

The baby should be placed with the mother as soon as possible after delivery to encourage bonding and to also allow for thermoregulation. However, it is best to ensure that the skin is dried as soon as possible as wet skin can allow a large proportion of heat loss via evaporation. In view of the large surface area to volume ratio, the losses are worse in babies. If the baby has irregular breaths at birth, gentle stimulation and clearing the airways may be enough to improve the condition of the baby and masks may be unnecessary. However, if the baby does not respond or meconium is seen in the pharynx/larynx, intubation with suction may be required.

32 T, T, T, T, T
Twenty-five per cent also follow abortion either spontaneous or induced. The success rate of treatment decreases to 40–75% when metastatic disease is present.

33 F, F, F, T, F
Risk of fetal lacerations is around 2%. Risk of postoperative infection is around 8%. Risk of urinary tract injury is around 0.1%. Risk of post-natal depression is not significantly higher than after vaginal delivery.

National Institute for Health and Clinical Excellence. *Caesarean Section: NICE guideline 13*. London: NIHCE; 2004. www.nice.org.uk/guidance/CG013

34 T, T, F, T, F
PID may lead to an increase in ectopic pregnancies and tubal infertility in the long term. Antibiotic prophylaxis with TOP helps reduce this. There is also a possible small increase of both preterm birth and future miscarriages. However the Royal Australian and New Zealand College of Obstetrics and Gynaecology (RANZCOG) in its TOP guidance states that the evidence does not support an association between termination of pregnancy and ectopic pregnancy.

RANZCOG. *Termination of Pregnancy: a resource for health professionals*. Melbourne: RANZCOG; 2005. www.ranzcog.edu.au/womenshealth/pdfs/Termination-of-pregnancy.pdf

35 T, T, F, T, T
There are few reasons why breast feeding should be limited and these are mainly due to serious illness such as HIV, TB, cancer, having chemotherapy and serious metabolic disorders in the baby. Previously, it had been thought that babies with phenylketonuria should not be breastfed to ensure a low phenylalanine intake; however, more recent studies have disputed this. The benefits are multifold and breast feeding should be encouraged as much as possible.

Motzfeldt K, Lilje R. Breastfeeding in phenylketonuria. *Acta Paediatr Suppl.* 1999; **88**(432): 25–7.

36 T, T, F, F, T

Other treatments include avoiding carbohydrates, limiting alcohol and caffeine, light therapy (with a bright white light via a face mask), red clover, transdermal oestradiol plus progestogens, citalopram on days 15–28, GnRH analogues and tibolone, or continuous combined low dose HRT and finally bilateral oophorectomy with or without hysterectomy plus HRT.

www.pms.org.uk

37 T, T, T, T, T

Infections can be either congenital or acute and thus can cause jaundice at any time. Metabolic, endocrine and genetic disorders can all cause prolonged jaundice. However, it is essential to rule out extra-hepatic biliary atresia in any neonate with prolonged jaundice, as swift surgical treatment could prevent cirrhosis and the need for liver transplantation.

38 F, T, F, F, T

Blood loss may be dark or fresh; other symptoms of ectopic pregnancy include shoulder tip pain as well as pain on urination or defecation, and fainting. Always think of ectopic if abdominal pain +/- bleeding. A cornual pregnancy is where the embryo implants into the interstitial rather than the extra-uterine part of the tube. The mortality rate is 1 in 50 compared to 1 in 3000 with other ectopic pregnancies as bleeding can be sudden and catastrophic.

39 T, F, T, T, F

The Brandt-Andrews method decreases the risk of uterine inversion; it involves uterine guarding and elevation, while providing cord traction during the third stage of labour. Management may include halothane anaesthetic to relax the uterus while warm saline is used under hydrostatic pressure into the vagina. Once resolved, ergometrine is administered to prevent further haemorrhage.

40 T, F, T, T, T

Chlamydia trachomatis is the most common curable STI in Britain. The National Chlamydia Screening programme started in 2003. A first-catch urine sample is required from both men and women, using ligase chain reaction/polymerase chain reaction in diagnosis. Asymptomatic infection can clear spontaneously.

www.bashh.org.uk

Index